The New
Get Back Into Your
Jeans Diet

The **New**
Get Back Into Your
Jeans Diet

MONICA GRENFELL

PAN BOOKS

First published 1999 by Pan Books
as *Get Back Into Your Jeans Diet*

This revised edition published 2003 by Pan Books
an imprint of Pan Macmillan Ltd
Pan Macmillan, 20 New Wharf Road, London N1 9RR
Basingstoke and Oxford
Associated companies throughout the world
www.panmacmillan.com

ISBN 978-0-330-41284-1

Exercise photographs by Lesley Howling

9 8 7 6 5 4 3 2

A CIP catalogue record for this book is available from
the British Library.

Typeset by SetSystems Ltd, Saffron Walden, Essex
Printed and bound in Great Britain by
Mackays of Chatham plc, Chatham, Kent

Visit **www.panmacmillan.com** to read more about all our books and to buy
them. You will also find features, author interviews and news of any author
events, and you can sign up for e-newsletters so that you're always first to hear
about our new releases.

Contents

Acknowledgements

This book is dedicated to my two wonderful sons, Michael and James Lavers, who are always so supportive and encouraging.

I would also like to thank all the people who took part in the diet testing and Tesco Stores plc for their help in supplying food information.

My particular gratitude goes to Gordon Wise at Pan Macmillan for his patience, enthusiasm, diplomacy, energy and skill as my editor, and for making it all such a pleasure.

Advice to the Reader

Before following any dietary or exercise advice contained in this book it is recommended that you consult your doctor if you suffer from any health problems or special conditions, or are in any doubt as to its suitability.

Monica's Mailbag

Let me know how you are getting on, tell me what problems you have and share with me how successful you have been getting back into your jeans! Email me at www.monicagrenfell.co.uk or write to me at:

Monica's Mailbag, PO Box 58 Oxon OX12 9BS

If you'd like a reply, please enclose a stamped self-addressed envelope.

Foreword

When I first wrote this book, in 1997, I could not have predicted how different life would become, so quickly. We all use computers and e-mail now. I'm not a slave to the internet, but I know how easy it would be. Satellite TV is everywhere. Basically, our bottoms are spreading, and getting back into those jeans is becoming more of a struggle than ever!

So much has changed, so fast, it was necessary to revise this diet and I have made it easier to follow. Even in these few years, people's attitudes have moved away from cooking and many people buy their meals pre-packaged. Salads, for example, are bought ready prepared but I would rather you ate a prepared salad than not eat salad at all. Soya milk and wheat-free diets have become more popular than I could have imagined and I wanted the diet to include them. But, somewhere along the line, for all the huge amount of diet advice out there, people are still gaining weight or failing to lose it. To combat this worrying trend, I have developed a new way of looking at the nutrients in our diets, and have come up with the concept of the carbogram.

There is nothing new about counting carbohydrates. Low-carbohydrate diets have dominated the scene for a couple of decades, but I have always found it impossible to exist on one. I believe there is a simple way of managing food intake so weight problems become a thing of the past. Yes, easy to trot out, but this time it's true. Manage carbohydrates and proteins in a realistic way, by matching energy output to input and you've got it cracked.

And you'll lose an astonishing amount of weight! With *The New Get Back Into Your Jeans Diet* I have taken away a lot of foods and meals you are unlikely to eat, and concentrated on the basics: what you need for health, what you need for appetite control and what you need for weight loss. The result is a brand-new, twenty-first-century approach to dieting which really works.

Don't listen to anybody who trots out that old line about diets not working. They do. I have dieted most of my life and never felt deprived, so read on and enjoy your diet. You're going to get back into those jeans and feel elegant, confident and beautiful – *I promise*!

Introduction

The Keys To Getting Back Into Your Jeans

Wouldn't you just love to be able to get back into your favourite jeans by this time next month? Or be a dress size smaller? Wouldn't we all! Well, with this plan you can – and you'll also discover that this is the last diet you'll ever need. I have written books on the best diet for a flatter stomach – *5 Days to a Flatter Stomach* – and the best diet for beauty – *Fabulous in a Fortnight* – and now I am going to give you the most successful diet I have ever devised – the ultimate weight-loss plan, whether you use it for a quick fix or to get you started on a whole new life of slimness.

This diet is foolproof. You're going to go down one dress size in a month, and you're going to feel sensational. If you can add up a column of figures you can lose weight successfully, just like the hundreds of elegant, glamorous women I advise every year. The old days of feeling washed-out, hungry and eating second-rate food are over. The past few decades have been littered with faddy diets, diets which ban a huge range of foods, diets which restrict fat or protein, or combinations of foods, diets which have had you lying awake half the night, hungry – and worst of all, diets which just didn't do anything for you. Well, on this diet you'll eat great food and still lose weight.

This is not a cosy plan which has you sitting back while I tell you what to do. I don't preach, but nor do I fool you that it is easy to be slim. It takes effort, and your input needs to be pretty high for the next month. But it's worth it. This is a campaign:

you're going to grit your teeth and go for it, and once you've gone down a size you can carry on and lose another. There's an exercise plan and records to keep (see pages 90 and 61–3), but that's the beauty of it – you can't go wrong because *you* are in the driving seat.

I have called this book *The New Get Back Into Your Jeans Diet* because experience tells me that most of us see weight loss in terms of wanting to regain a certain image. It's not just your body which bothers you, but how you look in your clothes. You've probably got fond memories of times when you felt good and looked good, and those memories are usually linked to clothes. They may have been your wedding dress, a special suit or your bikini, but they stay in your wardrobe as a benchmark. Gaining weight or losing your figure can mean more than just throwing out a few clothes which have become too tight. It can mean losing your identity. 'I just want to get back into those jeans!' has become such a familiar cry from my clients and the people who write to me that I decided to make it the title of this book. It also helps to point out that a good diet should be for *everybody* – I have as many letters from men as from women on the subject of weight loss and fitness, and most men are just as concerned about their health and appearance as women.

Mind you, weight loss is only part of the story. We all want to look *good* in our clothes and that means not just less fat, but toned muscles too. You might have lost half a stone, but what's happened to your stomach? And can you really bare your thighs on the beach, slim as they are?

You talk about losing your figure and wanting to get it back. Your figure is as much a part of your personality as the colour of your hair or your name. You own it. Size and shape are two of your main defining features. They matter, and in this book I am going to tell you how you can learn to shape up for good.

Men Don't Fall For Our Fat Ratios

In *5 Days to a Flatter Stomach* I pointed out that men don't fall for women's 'fat ratios', whatever slimming magazines might have us believe. A good figure and bags of confidence are what get you noticed. No one looks at you across a crowded room and thinks, 'She looks like she weighs nine stone, so she's the one for me.' They either like what they see – or they don't. If you feel awful being a size or two larger than you should be, you'll probably lack that crucial confidence. What I'm going to help you to do in this book is to regain your confidence.

But That's All About Losing Weight, Surely?

If you've weight to lose, yes, but you might be happy with your weight and unhappy with your shape. Most people have one bit of them which is out of step with conventional clothes' sizes, and if you sit down all day you're likely to have poor muscle tone. Other people need to lose a lot of weight before they can even consider exercising. I know one very large woman who can't walk more than one hundred metres without feeling shattered, so her first priority is to get her weight down.

Take the long view. You may have been a size 10 once. You're simply on the first rung of the ladder to getting back down to it. But start now, and make it a job that you want to do well.

Will There Be A Lot Of Exercise?

Up to a point. If you're the type of person who is well used to your nightly fix of aerobics, this will be a doddle. However, if you're never seen out of your armchair after 7 p.m., it'll be a shock. But likely as not you need to make exercise more of a permanent fixture in your life anyway; it shouldn't be something you 'fit in'. But nor do I want it to be something you endure or which bores you rigid.

One of the secrets of weight control lies in re-programming your body to expect a certain amount of food and exercise, so a commitment to the exercise programme, together with the food plan, is a must. Weight fluctuations will be a thing of the past once you understand that exercise isn't just a way of 'working off' what you've eaten. When you get to the section on 'homeostasis', this will make more sense (see pages 31–3).

Nobody was ever sorry because they went for a walk. Nobody ever felt worse for a stretch. Try to adopt the attitude that it's a necessary part of your goal. You can achieve a lot with diet, but it won't improve your shape.

I've made it simple for you by mapping out a realistic exercise programme which most people can manage. Your goals are clearly set out so that you know when you've done enough.

No time for exercise? I don't believe you. Everybody has twenty-four hours in a day, and we all have more time than our grandmothers. If you have a washing machine, you have time. If you have a car, you have time. If you ever sit for more than an hour each day watching television, you have time. If you value your figure, want to start afresh and make something of yourself, then you must *make* time. And I hate to say this, but *you* put the weight on in the first place. Eating less takes no time at all, and all the time you save from eating less can be spent in going for a walk! You'll never regret it.

I'm not talking about a vigorous regime which has you getting out of bed at five in the morning for fifty press-ups. And I'm not going to suggest that you leave the car at home and walk three miles in the rain just to lose half a pound. Yet if big thighs are your problem, they aren't going to disappear simply by wishing them away. Leg lifts and bottom squeezes, stomach crunches, waist whittlers and hamstring curls, oblique twists and hip stretches are all part of my daily repertoire of exercises that keep my clients toned and trim and admired by all their friends. I'm not saying we enjoy it, but who enjoys sitting at the hairdresser's with chemicals spread all over their hair? Yet we'll put ourselves through that expense and inconvenience a thousand times if it makes us look good. That's how you must approach your exercise routine: it's worth it, and the pay-off comes later. That pay-off being when you ask the assistant to fetch you a smaller size, or you make it back into your jeans.

So What's The Secret About This Diet?

It's all about eating in line with your energy requirements. Carbohydrate foods like potatoes, rice, pasta, cakes, sugar, fruit and milk all provide energy, but we all take in more than we need for the task ahead. If you are really about to embark on a charity half-marathon tomorrow, by all means go ahead and have a spaghetti Bolognese tonight. On the other hand, if you have to spend the day on a 10-hour train journey, you need less. It sounds like plain old common sense, but the way most people stoke up with food, you'd think they were off to the North Pole, not working on their backsides in an office. I'm guilty of it too. So this diet is about looking at your carbohydrate intake and your food intake as a whole, and matching it to your energy output. Simple as that.

To slim successfully and stay slim, you have to eat less. Nothing amazing about that, but there are times for all of us when it seems well-nigh impossible to avoid food. I am not talking about restaurants where you can order whatever you like. Meals with relatives, friends or colleagues can be times when people have gone to a lot of trouble on your behalf and it is churlish to refuse to eat what they have cooked for you. The secret of this diet is that you are in control. You can save carbograms from your daily CarboRange of 120–150 units and then eat pretty well what everyone else does. On most diets, you might let yourself go for the night, eat too much and wake the next day full of guilt and regret, but this won't happen with carbograms. I have given examples on pages 124–5 of the sort of meals you can eat when you go out using your CarboRange. I don't recommend it for everyday eating, but once or twice a month is fine.

This isn't boring. People talk about feeling deprived, but surely you are already deprived? Deprived of nice clothes, deprived of the feeling of stripping down to your bikini, deprived of admiring looks and compliments? The alternative to doing this diet is staying as you are.

You will be limiting added sugar in your diet. Sugar is a scourge of modern life because you don't have any control over the amount added by manufacturers. Foods which are an amalgamation of elements, such as cakes, are also banned. Cakes have fat, carbohydrate and sugar in them, and a lot more besides. In one mouthful you are cramming in the same amount of calories as you'd get in a roast chicken dinner with three veg! So no cakes, biscuits or ready-meals are allowed on this diet, just wholesome, plain foods with very low calorie values.

You must restrict food intake. There's no easy way of doing this apart from willpower and I am going to give you all the motivation I can. You *will* succeed. Not only that, but your weight will remain steady for the rest of your life.

How Weight Loss Happens

I prefer to talk about fat loss: weight is the total weight of your body and you can lose weight without losing fat. For example, in a very hot climate, or after a sauna, you could emerge three to five kilos lighter, but you haven't lost fat and you wouldn't look any different (and within a couple of hours you would have gained the weight back again). *Fat* loss is achieved when there is a negative energy balance, meaning more calories (the units of energy we get from eating food) are being eaten than you are using in activity. The average person uses 1–2 calories a minute at absolute rest, then more calories per minute depending on whether you are walking, running, sitting and so on. On this diet, calories more or less take care of themselves because you are eating less. Proteins are naturally low in fat and this in turn lowers your calorie intake, and your carbogram choices are such that you can only have one or two of the higher-calorie foods or meals per day. The average calorie count for each day of this diet is 1,400 – the perfect number to achieve weight loss of about a kilo a week even if you did no exercise whatever. But as you will be exercising, expect to lose about a further half a kilo a week just by being active.

I've Been Watching My Fat Intake – What About That?

Watching fat intake seems to work for some people, but it's not the Holy Grail in itself. The nation eats less fat than it did sixty years ago, yet obesity is at an all-time high. Why is this? Then, people ate less food and therefore fewer calories, and they took more exercise. They also planned their week's menus and bought only what they needed, and not what took their fancy. You had to ask for items, unlike today when you trundle round the shelves and pick up whatever you want. It is better to monitor fat by eating less food, and to eat foods which don't contain fat, than to eat fat-reduced foods such as yoghurts, biscuits and cakes. My own informal research has shown that instead of forgoing biscuits and cakes, people are actually choosing the lower-fat variety, thereby eating more than they mean to. I get so many letters from people who say they are not losing weight on a 'low-fat foods' diet that I can only conclude that they are still eating too many calories.

Fat intake looks after itself on this diet because there is very little fat in basic foods. Since you only eat one or two protein foods – such as fish, eggs, nuts or meat – fat is automatically cut there too. Your only task is to keep records of your food intake for a month. After that, it will become second nature.

People often say that they don't want to be bothered with weighing out food portions and counting calories. Then, in the next breath, they talk of their despair about their weight. They say that they can't be bothered fiddling with food diaries, but they think nothing of spending an hour cooking, eating or bingeing on food which makes them ill. Fine then, stay as you are! I don't want to sound mean, but there's effort involved in achieving anything. If you've tried everything else and it hasn't worked, why not just give this a go? I have provided suggestions for all the menus for you (see pages 126–68). Stick with the main menus and devise all the permutations you like.

Counting By Carbograms

I call my method of carbohydrate counting 'carbograms'. Keeping carbohydrates within a sensible level is the key to weight loss. When you see how much of your carbogram budget can be spent on a bagel or a plate of pasta, you will want to save them for something more worthwhile. On the other hand, you might want a girls' night out, and decide to save up for one meal. That's fine.

When I was young, carbohydrates were seen as stodgy and fattening, and modern high-protein diets have reinforced this myth. It is easy to advise someone only to eat chicken or bacon or eggs or fish and to avoid bread, and disciples of these regimes say they work. Yes, they lose weight, but if you are hungry and the only thing you can eat is a chicken breast or a rasher of bacon, it's hardly likely that you're going to wait while you grill or fry or roast them first. True, you might have some cold chicken or a hard-boiled egg handy, but who craves cold chicken or a boiled egg? Bread can be grabbed. Crisps can be grabbed. Gradually the calories pile on as sandwiches are made or a pizza base gets its six toppings. It isn't the carbohydrates that cause the problems, but what you have with them. On their own, they are vital, essential, inexpensive and incredibly handy and convenient ways to feed yourself. Where would we all be without sandwiches?

Carbohydrates are your energy source. No serious athlete, bodybuilder or dancer would dream of going on a protein-only diet. The energy from carbohydrates is stored in your muscles and liver as glycogen, and you can retain about 1,600 calories at any one time. Go over this number, especially in one meal, or by eating two meals within a couple of hours, and you start to store the excess calories as fat. By staying within a reasonable calorie range at each meal, you store them for use in the short-term and of course, use them up in activity.

Even if you ate nothing else, protein foods on their own can make you fat. Fish has calories. Meat has calories. Indeed, a fillet of salmon has more calories than a medium-sized jacket potato and these calories either eventually get used or they don't. If they don't, you store fat. You only have to think of the stout figures in Dickensian novels who ate a high meat diet and had no snacks or sweets, to realize that protein diets aren't all they are cracked up to be. Proteins are essential, but you need carbohydrates for a truly rounded, successful weight-loss diet.

Incidentally, I know countless people, some of them celebrities, who only practise protein diets for half the time. They'll sneakily demolish a slice of pizza when nobody's looking!

These are the amounts of protein, fat and carbohydrate needed by the average person:

carbohydrate:	120–150g
protein:	48g
fat:	70g (21g saturated)

Even on a reduced carbohydrate diet, you need about 120g per day. An extremely active person only needs a reduced calorie and carbohydrate diet if they have a weight problem – a *real* weight problem of more than 12 kilos or over 30 per cent body fat. If you are very active and slim, you won't be reading this book. But most people's perceptions of what active means are wildly different. An overweight person will often feel that normal activities are exhausting purely because their weight makes it so. If you're not used to walking, a one-mile walk to town can finish you off. People often tell me that they are always phenomenally hectic and they never stop, but I have followed such people around for a day and was dying to get going and do something! Feeling hassled can be draining. Being stressed can feel like a workout. People are quite amazed when their weight doesn't budge, or they lose a bit and then 'plateau', but they are probably still eating more than they think and not using up as many calories as they feel they are. The answer is to work with carbograms.

Counting Carbograms

I could not give carbogram values for every food item you are likely to eat, but most people get used to the meals that crop up time and again, and know their values automatically. Food labelling has been a great boon. If you are in any doubt about carbograms, look at the nutrition information panel on packaged goods – it should tell you all you need to know. It will also come up with a few surprises! Write down the items you eat most frequently and pin up a list on your fridge or wherever. Beans on toast, tuna salad, steak and chips – these are all quite normal meals and perfectly acceptable on the Jeans diet, but you need to know their carbogram values for your daily 'budget'. Starting on page 117 are the carbogram values for most of the everyday meals you are likely to want – there at a glance with each element separately valued.

Sugar

An important part of this diet is the restriction of added sugars. In the medical and dieting world not much has been made of the true part played by sugar – partly, I think, because it is not linked to any major disease. However, unlike fat, added sugar is one food for which your body has absolutely no need. The only reason it is added to food is to make it taste better, although it thereby encourages a 'sweet tooth' (and not very good ones, either!). Personally, I think this is terrible. Man isn't meant to eat sweet food, except for naturally sweet things, like fruit. By cutting out sugar, you will automatically reduce your calorie intake and gradually lose weight in a painless way. If you eat a diet that is rich in complex carbohydrates, control your portions and embark on an exercise plan, you will soon find that you can go for days without needing your old sugar 'fix'.

My Promise

Here is my promise to you if you continue this plan for a month:

- You will stop bingeing and craving food.
- You will never have fluctuating weight again.
- You will not wake up and step straight onto the scales.
- You will not worry about every mouthful, every social event and every pound.
- You will not care about your weight, only your size.

You are going to lose weight, go down a whole size and get back into those jeans. You will never look back! I really understand how to control weight. This is my ultimate weight-loss plan and I am confident of its success for you.

Back To Basics

Your Body Has A Mind Of Its Own

You can only begin to understand weight control when you can understand why you store fat in the first place. Forget fancy diets which say that you can't mix some foods, or tolerate others. Man is a hunter, designed with the ability to eat massive quantities of food in one go, as available, and to mix anything with everything, storing most of it as available energy and saving the excess as fat for harder times.

Today, despite the easy availability of fast food and little danger of starvation in developed countries, we are still the same animals, and eating more than we need means that we store fat. This is a perfectly normal human function. Some people wonder what's gone wrong when they start to gain weight. Nothing's wrong. Your body is simply doing what comes naturally with the fuel that it doesn't immediately need.

Mother Nature has only one thing on her mind – the survival of the species. However, what Nature doesn't know is that if you are a woman, you may have decided not to have children or you may have already completed your family. As far as your body knows, if you are fertile, you need stores of fat, regardless of any pregnancy. Fat stores are usually positioned around the hips, stomach and thighs. This is why women have greater trouble in losing fat from the lower body, although fat stores can be anywhere including the back, arms and chin!

Your body doesn't know that it isn't always going to have to sustain a pregnancy, or to hang on for a few days until the next

13

meal is available. So it still stores fat in case of need. But this doesn't mean that it doesn't know best. If you place your body under starvation conditions by crash dieting, or being on a continual diet of too few calories, you will be on a permanent seesaw of weight gain and weight loss. Later on in the book I will explain this in more detail. In the meantime, it is important that you understand the processes which govern our metabolisms.

Never put your body into 'starvation' mode by going for hours or days without sufficient food. Listen to its pleas for food and nourishment and act on the signals. Your body has a mind of its own. If you treat it badly, it will pay you back in terms of yo-yoing weight gain and loss, moodiness, irritability, depression and failure. Listen to your body: it deserves better than this.

My Foolproof Way To
Lasting Slimness

Does this sound familiar? For years, you've dieted without success. There's nothing you haven't tried. The result is always the same. During the first week you lose 2.25–3.75 kilos (5–8lb) and then you get stuck. Your friends seem to eat anything they like and still stay slim, never gaining so much as an inch or a pound. You tell yourself you know the reason why: you have a slow metabolism and other people just burn calories off faster than you do.

I'm afraid you're wrong. The correct reason for this is that you aren't active enough, and you probably eat more food than you think. You may not eat much, and you've probably been watching fat content rather than calories, but even a fat-less diet can be loaded with calories. In terms of energy burning, the key to weight loss is the calories. For example, a 98 per cent fat-free bagel has 235 calories and 43 carbograms. A teaspoon of jam, which is totally fat-free, has 70 calories and 10 carbograms. On a calorie-restricted diet these figures soon mount up to a calorie count that is well over your basic needs, and being just a few calories over the limit on a regular basis soon leads to the sort of weight gain that you find baffling. I get a lot of letters through my weekly Sunday magazine column which say exactly the same thing: 'I seem to have put on a stone in the past year and I don't know how. I'm eating the same as I always did, but the weight's creeping on.' It's very upsetting, but people don't realize how these little differences can add up to a big difference over time, especially if you aren't exercising.

What About Calories?

All foods have calories. A calorie is a unit of energy, and while some foods have more than others, even a lettuce leaf supplies a calorie. A nut has calories, so does fish or chicken, but they are almost totally carbohydrate-free. So you can't eat masses of them with gay abandon and expect your weight to melt away. It just doesn't happen like that.

I am spotlighting carbohydrates because they are the foods we all fall down on. I'd like to meet the person who sticks her hand in the fridge for some salmon. Or the person who dives into the petrol station, ravenous, gasping for liver and bacon. Convenience food deserves its name, but for some reason we find sweet, fatty foods more convenient than savoury, healthy ones; they're cooked, filled, dusted, iced, tossed in several tasty coatings and they go in the mouth a treat. This layering of flavours is the most tempting thing for the body because it has been shown in numerous studies that the more flavours there are, the more our appetites are stimulated. Junk food is everywhere. Calories call out to you from roadside kiosks to petrol stations to corner shops and even garden centres. Throwing 400 or even 600 calories down your throat and calling it a snack takes no more effort than getting out your purse. Pork pies, Cornish pasties and crisps are other favourites where the calorie intake far outweighs our needs, but they consist mainly of carbohydrates – with a lot of added fat – so by limiting them we automatically limit calories. Why? Because if the only things in your fridge you can eat are cold meat, eggs or salads, you are less likely to go mad on them or if you do, you are less likely to eat too many calories.

But If I'm Carbohydrate Counting, Will I Become A Carbohydrate 'Junkie'?

You certainly shouldn't. However, you might worry that once you start focusing on the carbohydrate content of food, you will be carrying around a carbohydrate reference book for the rest of your life. Don't worry. You will soon get to know roughly how many carbohydrates are contained in what sort of foods, and after a while it will become second nature. I bought a carbohydrate-counting mini computer a while ago, which told me how many carbohydrates I was burning in daily activities. At first I wore it all the time. I was so fascinated I couldn't take it off. How many carbohydrates was I burning off during my keep-fit class? How many carbohydrates were shed in that walk round the village? How many an hour at my word processor? After a while it got crazy. But I soon realized that most days evened out to about the same. I also found that I wasn't using as many carbohydrates as I thought I was, and I adjusted my food intake accordingly. You'll find you won't be counting carbohydrates for ever, because you won't need to.

Your Questions Answered

Why does my weight keep fluctuating, and why do I gain weight so easily?
I receive hundreds of letters every month, and I see dozens of clients. If there is one theme that recurs time and time again, this letter really says it all . . .

Please help me. I am twenty years old and have always been overweight. By July 1995 I weighed 11½ stone [69kg] which was the final straw. I started exercising and cutting down on snacks. My weight gradually fell and when I started university it kept on

falling because I began an aerobics class as well. By March 1997 I weighed 9st 4lb [56kg] and was a size 14.

I was looking and feeling great. There were several times when I had a binge, but due to the aerobics I managed to maintain that weight. Then during summer break this year, my weight went back up to 9st 12lb [59kg]. I was paranoid about the other weight returning and went on a stupid diet with a friend who advised me to eat only one 'healthy' meal a day and to exercise. I took this to an extreme in order to reach my goal of losing a stone [6kg] in a month. My daily food intake consisted of one bowl of cereal for breakfast, an apple for lunch and just boiled rice with vegetables in the evening. I also overdid it with the exercise, doing two hours every day. I felt very tired, but stuck to it. I was overjoyed at the end of the month when I weighed in at 8st 12lb [53kg] and took a size 10–12.

But from that day on I began bingeing. Sometimes I felt out of control, eating up to six slices of pizza with chips, cakes and chocolates in one sitting. To make up for this, I starved myself the next day.

Six months later, I weigh 10 stone [60kg]. I have been strict with myself, trying to allocate realistic lifetime targets that I can maintain even after weight loss. I go to aerobics three times a week, always walk around instead of driving and take the stairs wherever possible. I am a chocoholic but have resisted the temptation so far. I eat cereal for breakfast, fruit and a sandwich for lunch and have spicy foods in the evenings. I have been following this routine for the past three weeks but my weight has nonetheless increased to 10st 3lb [61.2kg].

I just don't understand where I am going wrong. At times I feel as if I am going mad. The first thing I think about before doing anything is how much I can eat and what to eat, and this obsession is driving me crazy. I can't seem to concentrate on anything. I just want to be 9 stone [54kg]. I have tried everything, but all the weight is on my stomach and 'love handles', and I have gone from a size 12 to a 14–16. Every time I set myself a target I find I just give up because it doesn't work any more. Please help me!

Anita, Glasgow

The problem here is essentially one of chaotic eating and a lack of control. In Back to Basics (see pages 13–14), I talked about the logic behind nature's need to store fat. However, in the normal course of events, nature is not so stupid as to store so much fat that it slows you down. Regular, frequent eating reassures your brain that your body is always going to be fed. The point is to control the intake.

I can best describe the impact of chaotic eating on your body by asking you to picture a parallel scenario which you probably wouldn't contemplate: try sleeping for three hours tomorrow morning and two hours the following afternoon, then skip the following night's sleep altogether and make up for it by having twelve hours the next day. Then deprive yourself of all sleep for a solid three days. How do you think you would feel? Exactly.

People who regularly have erratic sleeping habits get out of sorts and find their bodily functions become out of step. Yet many of us, including Anita, expect our bodies to cope with constantly changing eating patterns: piles of pizza, chips and chocolate followed by a day of nothing; wild aerobics for three weeks with calories severely restricted, followed by mountains of food and no exercise at all. In the middle of this nightmare Anita expects her body to lose weight. Well, the body doesn't actually respond to a day without food by shedding – or using up – fat. On a strict diet like the one that Anita followed for a month, hours were passing without her consuming any food at all. In this situation the body's only response is to shut down its systems to save as many calories as possible, which is one reason why she felt so tired. The body can store between 1,600 and 2,000 calories at a time, which are generally used up in the course of a day, but as these stores become depleted you begin to feel weak and lethargic.

On this kind of diet what you won't do, however, is to use fat. Yes, Anita lost weight, but at least half of that was glycogen and water, two of her body's most vital components. Her actual fat loss, I suspect, was very little and it was inevitable that she not only gained back the weight, but also binged madly because she missed eating, and her body was worried that it might never see food again. In such circumstances the metabolism slows down considerably to save fuel and this is why weight is always regained at such an alarming rate.

You must get into a routine! Lack of routine is one of the main reasons why people become fat. When I say 'chaotic' eating, I don't mean grabbing a sandwich for lunch, or occasionally skipping breakfast. I mean dieting and bingeing like Anita. A binge is eating for the sake of it, saying 'to hell with it' as you clear up after guests and finish off the trifle and cheese just because it's there. A binge is what you feel you need when you've been on a diet but have broken it by having a slice of cake, and you then hate yourself. You feel guilty, so you buy a chocolate bar on your way home and eat it because you might as well. You probably have it in the back of your mind that you'll start afresh tomorrow, so you might as well eat while you are still in the mood.

Bingeing is a frame of mind. It comes on when you have deprived your body of nutrients, and chemically it is screaming out and sending instinctive messages to the brain. Bingeing happens when you feel the damage is so bad, you might as well add to it. It is one of the causes of weight gain and is brought on by chaotic eating.

Anita will beat her problem when she learns to take a longer view. She must start now and get her confidence up. Anita must stop weighing herself constantly, start to eat four times a day and give it three months at least. If she follows the advice in this book, her weight problems will never return.

On this plan you will say goodbye to bingeing and starving by following a frequent-eating, carbohydrate-loaded diet. You'll get back into your old jeans by next month and never look back!

Why do I get food cravings?

Food cravings are your body's cry for help. To understand them, imagine a really raging thirst. What does it make you want to do? You have to have a drink. Now, think about being really cold. What does this make you want to do? You put on extra layers of clothes. And what if you are terribly hot? You take off some of your clothes or go somewhere to cool down. Sensations, such as thirst, are hard to describe and you don't always know where they come from, but they are irresistible. They make you do exactly what you must in order to prevent a life-threatening situation – in this case, dehydration. Hunger, cold and heat are also life-threatening situations and your body forces you to do something about them by providing a sensation to which you respond. Feeling an irresistible urge to eat is the same kind of force. Your body needs nutrients which you are not giving it and it therefore provides the urge. It is as simple as that.

One of the most common cravings is for magnesium, another is for fat. It may not surprise you to learn that both of these are contained in chocolate! People who are on strict diets are very likely missing their magnesium intake, so they are the most likely to binge out on chocolate and fatty foods, thus keeping the crave–binge–starve cycle going. I should also add here that chocolate contains caffeine, and caffeine is highly addictive.

People who talk about getting their daily chocolate 'fix' are, in fact, craving caffeine, as well as magnesium and fat. What's unfortunate is that chocolate also contains a lot of calories per bar. If you're in any doubt that fat is a major source of craving for the human body, ask yourself when you last saw someone bingeing on broccoli, or chicken liver or fresh crab meat? How about lentils and tomatoes? We all know the jokes about pregnant women's cravings, but under normal circumstances we just don't binge on those foods; instead, we binge on mountains of buttered toast, whole pizzas, chips and chocolate gateaux. It happens most of all when a diet has been too low in fat and calories due to a desire to lose weight in the fastest possible time. *Fatless diets cause cravings and binges.*

The other reason why we binge is low blood sugar. If you insist on skipping breakfast and you eat very little during the day, you will crave sugar. Sugar enters the bloodstream very quickly and provides instant relief from tiredness and hunger, but the downside is that it triggers off what is known as the 'insulin response'. Insulin is secreted into your body to prevent your blood sugar from going dangerously high, but it also provides too much in anticipation of a further meal. If a meal doesn't come along, your blood sugar will be low and this results in a feeling of weakness and lethargy.

The way to beat irresistible cravings is to eat regularly. However, you have a weight problem which is bothering you and food is obviously the culprit, so is it right to say that you 'need never feel hungry' on a diet?

I don't believe so. It was a dislike of hunger and a liking for food which got you to where you are now, and hunger is not bad in itself. For example, if you are going out for a special meal in the evening, might you not enjoy it all the more for having worked up a real hunger for it? There's a difference between being hungry because you're trying not to eat – which is *bad* – and being nicely hungry for your next meal, and this is what you must learn on your new plan. Don't listen to people who tell you you need never do without your favourite foods or be hungry if you are to lose weight successfully: you do. But you are doing it sensibly, retraining yourself and developing your most precious asset – WILLPOWER! So start now, establish a routine which fits in with your life and stick to it. And follow these golden rules:

- If you have a big meal one evening, *don't* get up the next day and skip breakfast and lunch to make up for it. Eat your meals as you would have done normally so that your body learns to trust you. Knowing that you will have to eat the next day may also stop you from overeating in the first place.
- Don't starve yourself all day just because you have a special event to go to in the evening and are thinking that you are bound to overeat. Have your usual meals. If you suspect a high-calorie feast is in the offing, compensate for this by cutting down on portions at your usual meals, such as having one piece of toast instead of two, a salad instead of soup for lunch, etc. *But don't eat nothing at all!*

You will find that regular eating banishes cravings. If you are a lover of 'fattening' foods, remember that *no* foods are fattening in themselves. It is the calorie and carbogram content that matters.

Why is my friend so slim when we both eat the same things?
This has a lot to do with your genetic tendency to store fat in certain parts of the body. My family, for example, all store fat in the upper body which leads to double chins and spare tyres! The only saving grace we have is that we hardly ever get fat legs or bottoms. A common mistake, though, is to believe that a tendency means an *inevitability*; it doesn't. Never mind that

your aunties and your cousin and your three sisters all have fat thighs, it doesn't mean that you will too. My family don't all have double chins, but that's the first place where my weight goes.

We all envy other people's tiny waists or thin thighs, but the fact is that no one was born with a God-given ability to eat just anything they like and not gain weight. If your friend eats a lot and is slim, it simply means she's using her fuel and you aren't. There's always a reason. Look at the section on calorie burning and exercise (see pages 90–93), and you will see how changes in ordinary everyday tasks (such as washing a car instead of going through the car wash) can make a lot of difference to your calorie burning.

Which foods are fattening and which ones aren't?

No food is fattening and no food is slimming. It's all down to how much you eat of it. I have already talked about calories and cravings, and the fact is that if you are a 'chocoholic' you *should* include some chocolate in your daily diet. Remember, though, that chocolate is not as healthy as fruit, and the fruit should be there too!

Fat yields nine calories per gram, as opposed to protein and carbohydrate which have four calories per gram, hence you can eat more of these without gaining weight. Simply remember that all foods have the potential to cause weight gain if you eat more than your body needs.

Too much sugar makes you feel lack-lustre and irritable. Sugar causes the 'insulin response' as explained earlier (see page 22), but many people respond to that by having *more* sugar! Being fed a constant supply of sweets, chocolate bars and fizzy drinks without pausing for a square meal, your appetite is constantly dampened and you don't give your body the chance to get properly hungry for a really good meal. Blood-sugar levels swing wildly and the effect on your moods can be dramatic. Just ask any diabetic!

My next ban is on junk food. Too many additives are simply not good for you or your digestive system. Pure, fresh food is a *must*. If you take a little time to prepare food, this also means that you may think twice about what you eat instead of just cramming in something you've microwaved in a minute.

If you want to lose weight, cut down on portions. Ration yourself to specific weights and amounts. Don't just snack, even on endless amounts of fruit and vegetables, just because you think they're not fattening. Get into overall good habits with food – it is not your enemy!

How can I stop picking in the evening?

You don't need to. You may not believe it, but evening eating is not outlawed on my diet, nor should it be. There is a lot of rubbish talked about late eating going to fat, and it's a fallacy. I have already talked a lot about routine and if your routine is one of evening eating, then carry on. Remember that many people, such as professional actors and dancers, not to mention shift workers, have to eat late. They aren't all fat!

However, there's a world of difference between 'picking' in the evening and eating an evening meal, and you shouldn't be doing both. Picking at food when you are not hungry comes down to basic boredom and habit, and the best way to stop this is to save your meal for as late as possible (within reason), and to make sure that it is not too fatty, too sweet or too large. For example, it is not a good idea to have a main meal *and* a pudding, unless that pudding is fruit or a light mousse-type dessert.

In an ideal world you should make breakfast your biggest meal, your midday meal a reasonable size and your evening meal very small – but life isn't always like that! Most of us race around in the day and snatch a sandwich if we're lucky, and what could be nicer than relaxing in the evening with a good meal and possibly a glass of wine? It's not quite the same thing, gazing over the candlelight at a ham sandwich! Here are the golden rules about late eating:

- Don't have a full roast and two veg. Meat takes about eight hours to pass through the system and you won't sleep well if your body is working hard to digest it.
- Don't eat fried food, or food which is too sweet, late at night.
- Make room for a late snack by eating a lot less earlier on.
- Try not to eat later than 10 p.m.
- Do not have heavy sauces, such as cheese sauce, white sauce or sauce with cream in it. Pasta sauces made with vegetables and tomato sauce are lighter and more digestible.
- An ideal meal would be potatoes with fish and vegetables or salad. If you just want a snack, try toast or cereal with fresh fruit.

The best way to manage evening eating is to exercise first. Go to a fitness class or the gym, or have a brisk walk or run on summer evenings. Perhaps you might spend the evening gardening? All these activities are ideal for evening eaters because the body uses food more effectively when it is taken *after* exercise when your muscles are restocking themselves. I think of it being like bare shelves in a supermarket after the Christmas rush. You need to stock up again quickly, ready for the next rush of customers!

How can I raise a slow metabolism?
How do you know that your metabolism is slow? Is it because you gain weight so easily? And just what is metabolism anyway?

It is the rate at which your body burns its fuel and it is rather like an engine. A Rolls-Royce uses a lot of fuel because it is so big and heavy, but a Mini uses little fuel because it is small and has an uncomplicated engine. Your metabolism depends on the following:

- your age
- your weight
- your gender
- the amount you eat
- the amount of muscle you have
- the amount of exercise you take

Let us look at each of these in turn:

Your Age

Your body weight is a mixture of everything contained inside you, so it won't surprise you to learn that putting on weight doesn't necessarily mean that you've gained fat. Weight is also muscle and your metabolism is muscle-driven.

If you're gradually losing muscle because you're getting older – and who isn't? – your metabolic rate will also decrease. It isn't a lot over a year, but it starts from the age of about twenty-five. By the time you've reached forty you're possibly just beginning to notice what started years ago, and it's called 'middle-age spread' – fat stored around the middle which our slowed-down metabolism isn't dealing with any more. If you add to that a natural tendency to slow down as you get older, to become more placid and less easily upset, or maybe the children have left home so there's less running around, or perhaps you've been promoted to a more desk-bound job, or retired so you aren't working at all and/or you have fewer money worries, then it can seem as though you've suddenly gained weight at the age of forty-five. In fact, the process began about twenty years ago.

Remember, ageing is not just something that happens to people who are older than you are. *Even if you are eighteen, you are still ageing. Take steps before it becomes a problem.* The secret of keeping abreast of metabolism changes is to *increase the amount of exercise you do for muscle strength*, thereby keeping up your muscle size, and to *increase the amount of aerobic activity you carry out.*

Your Weight

I have already talked about the difference between a Mini and a Rolls-Royce when it comes to fuel consumption. When you weigh a lot, your body needs a lot more fuel to keep it going. If you weigh very little, your resting metabolic rate will be a lot lower.

Your Gender

Men have a higher resting metabolic rate than women because they have a greater proportion of muscle on their bodies. It doesn't necessarily mean that a man has a higher capacity for exercise, and a man who sits at a desk all day will have an inferior endurance to a woman who keeps fit on a regular basis. But on the whole, women do have 80 per cent less active muscle than men and they store more body fat. It won't be much comfort to women for them to know that in the event of starvation, they will survive longer than men, but the fact remains that the higher proportion of muscle in men means that their metabolism is slightly higher.

The Amount You Eat

The body does a lot of amazing things in a week:

- Your heart beats more than 700,000 times.
- You breathe more than 121,000 times.
- Your stomach produces almost five litres of digestive juices.
- Your entire outer skin cells are replaced.
- Your hair grows about two millimetres.
- 1,750 gallons of blood passes through your kidneys.

And to think that some people do this on a diet of next to nothing!

All these functions – and many more – happen even if you are asleep, and on top of them you have your daily life with its stresses and strains. We all have what is called a 'Basal Metabolic Rate' (BMR). This is the number of calories needed to keep all your basic processes going, even if you were to lie in bed all day doing nothing at all. It's the reason why a person still needs to be fed, even if he is in a coma. Your BMR depends on how big a body you have and how much muscle you have, and it's fair to calculate your resting BMR at about a calorie – or just under a calorie – for every minute of the twenty-four-hour day.

The process of eating *raises* the body's metabolic rate because digesting food requires energy. If you eat frequently, there is always something going through your system so that it won't shut down to starvation levels. When I was at school, there was an old wives' tale that we teenage girls used to trot out about a boiled egg being worth 'minus' calories because it took more calories to digest than it actually contained. I think it was probably a bit of an exaggeration, but even so there was a grain of common sense in the theory. Certain foods require a lot of energy to be broken down by the body, and hard-boiled eggs, high-fibre foods and meat are just three of them. The basic point is that digestion uses energy and starving yourself requires none.

The Amount Of Muscle On Your Body

You can weigh 54 kilos (9 stone) of muscle or 54 kilos (9 stone) of fat. Most of us are a mixture of both. Naturally slim people often eat little and take no exercise, and as they get older their lack of muscle tone not only leads to weakness and injury, but also weight gain. By keeping good muscle tone your metabolism is raised and you can enjoy food without gaining weight.

The Amount Of Exercise You Take

The best type of exercise for increasing your metabolic rate is muscular-strength work. Next comes aerobic exercise. Exercise should be vigorous and last for more than forty-five minutes. The general medical advice is to do a minimum of twenty minutes' hard exercise three times a week for health purposes, but if you are young you can easily manage forty-five minutes. And the best reason for exercising vigorously is that it uses up your body's glycogen stores which are then replenished after activity. It should take only two minutes for your heart rate to recover after strenuous exercise, but your blood pressure and metabolic rate stay high for up to two hours afterwards, which makes it the best time to eat. Your metabolic rate is also higher, even when resting, if you have been working at improving the tone of your muscles.

A final word about exercise. Talk about muscle–fat ratios, strength training, resistance training and endurance can be off-putting if you're new to exercise. It sounds as if you'll be weight lifting and running marathons, and it conjures up pictures of you sweating away in a gym or squeezing your hips into a tight

Lycra leotard! Well, it doesn't have to be any of these. The activity can be anything from combing your hair to vacuuming the carpet to pruning the roses. Strength training is anything that requires muscular strength, such as heaving furniture, digging the garden or cycling. Endurance is anything you can do for a long time, like going for a couple of hours' walk. If there is one message that I want to get across it is that exercise is anything you want it to be, and it needn't cost anything.

Why Have I Suddenly Gained All This Weight?

Many people who have been slim all their lives ask me this when they find that their 'normal' weight seems to have increased. If you've never needed to worry about your weight, it can be very upsetting. You're following the same routine and living the same life, yet the weight is piling on – or is it? When I investigate clients who complain about sudden weight gain, it's usually happened over a long period of maybe a year. It's all down to a process called 'homeostasis', which is the body's ability to regulate itself over a period of weeks and months, rather than hours or days. It is the body's overall ideal functioning state of balance and applies to all your functions – your salt–fluid balance, for example, or your sugar levels, or your hormone levels. Your general weight is also subject to this balance, so although most of us fluctuate by a few kilos either way, there is usually a mid-point at which your body is happiest.

When your weight is usually steady, a weekend's heavy eating won't make any difference at all. If you starve yourself for a day, then it won't make any difference either, and any weight loss is soon regained. We all know that it is possible for the body to lose a lot of weight very quickly, say in the case of a jockey or boxer who has to register at a certain weight to qualify for competition. I know of one jockey who 'lost' 4.5

kilos (10lb) in weight in just four hours by taking diuretics tablets which made him lose fluids rapidly, but this wasn't his 'true' weight, of course. (It's also not at all good for your body's system, and I'd advise against taking diuretics as part of any weight-loss plan.) As soon as his race was over and he had had a few cups of tea his body retained them and his weight shot back up again by 4.5 kilos. This is homeostasis (see below) working! The body has remarkable ability to maintain balance, and you've got to work with it. These extreme measures make no difference to your shape and size, so if you want to start afresh, get slim – and get back into those jeans – you need a different approach. You need *routine, regular meals* and *exercise*.

The Miracle Of Homeostasis

Here's how homeostasis works in practice. Say you were used to a ten-minute walk to work and back every day for years and you gave up work to have a baby. A major part of your routine will have been altered. It may have seemed like nothing in comparison with all the other changes, but twenty minutes of walking, five days a week for forty-eight weeks a year, is eighty hours of walking. It takes 24,000 calories of fuel to achieve this, doubtless mopping up a good amount of your excess intake! On top of that, what if you used to have just coffee for elevenses every day and now you have two biscuits with it? Again, it doesn't seem much for one day, but if this becomes a routine then you have added 500 calories a week or 26,000 calories a year. With the loss of the outlet of 24,000 calories and the additional 26,000 calories, this equates to six kilos (a whole stone) in weight!

The point is, having the odd couple of biscuits won't change your weight, and forgoing your daily walk for a few days won't make any difference either. However, the problem arises when you give up one routine which is firmly embedded and take on another. Weight 'creeps up' on us because we don't take these little changes in food and exercise into account – but your body does. Your body becomes programmed to your routine and will stick with what it knows, unless you start to reprogramme it with a new routine. Many young mothers find that their weight changes for the worse when they stay at home and they find it baffling because life is so hectic. It is also demoralizing to feel unattractive and fat, but keeping busy is not the same as being active. Physical activity is what burns calories.

You let weight creep up on you by not paying attention to the little things like exercise and the odd cake or biscuit. Soon you have relaxed your standards and 'let yourself go'. The good news is that the process also works in reverse. This diet plan will get you back into good habits and hopefully make you aware of how to balance what you are eating in terms of extra food and how that relates to activity for the rest of your life.

Influencing homeostasis is a way of setting a computer programme. As we know, people who have been used to crash dieting find that whenever they start to eat normally again, they gain weight. This is natural, but if you wait and let your new programme lodge itself into your system, your weight will soon fall again. Exercise is subject to this control too and when you start a new exercise programme it may take a few weeks before you notice a real difference. *But it will happen!* Just sit tight, stick with the plan, watch the carbograms and let nature take its course.

Getting Back Into Your Jeans

How Does This Diet Work?

Let's just recap on where we've got to so far. Weight problems and failing to manage your weight at the end of a diet are caused by:

- eating too many calories
- eating too many carbograms
- eating chaotically – 'grabbing' what's there
- having unhealthy snacks in the house
- eating between meals
- lack of willpower

Here is how you are going to deal with these challenges:

1 *Eating too many calories and carbograms*
Calculate your carbogram level and stick with it. You can spread the carbograms out over three meals, but you MUST have some carbohydrates with breakfast, maybe a portion of cereal and milk or two slices of toast with an egg. You will find it hard to exceed the calories you need even if you aren't counting them, because the size of your meals is automatically limited by the type of carbograms you can eat. High-calorie foods tend to be the ones full of sugar or fat, and on the *Get Back Into Your Jeans Diet* there are no sweet or fatty meals. The only exception to the calorie rule might be if you ate a particularly large steak or a double helping of salmon, for example, but I think it unlikely that you could manage to get

through either of these protein foods without a lot of carbo-hydrates to make them more palatable!

2 Eating chaotically

Chaotic eating means reaching into your office drawer for a sandwich, eating in the street, eating while you're preparing food and eating at odd times. This leads to weight gain. *The only way to successfully beat the problem is to retrain yourself.* It sounds harsh and you probably feel as though you're being treated like a child, but trust me. On this plan you'll be fixing mealtimes and sticking to them. You'll schedule everything, even your snacks or cups of tea. Believe it or not, although you'll start by thinking about your next meal and gasping for the next snack, your frustration won't last. You've probably got an unbalanced approach to food right now which is why those jeans or that dress won't fit, but in the long run, your new habits will bring you a lot of happiness – and clothes that fit!

3 Failing to plan meals

In the hustle and bustle of daily life, you probably lurch into a supermarket and wait for inspiration to strike. I've done it myself. The biggest problem about this approach is that it leads to what I call the 'pineapple syndrome'. This is an old joke in our household. Many years ago, I bought a pineapple because it was reduced in price. I was in a hurry, I hadn't a clue what we were going to eat, and I was casting around the shop for inspiration. I shoved the pineapple in the fridge and then forgot all about it. Two weeks later I found it and a stab of guilt flashed through me as I fought my desire to chuck it out straight away. It's good food, I thought. I'm sure I can do something with it.

Half an hour and five recipe books later, I settled on a Pineapple Upside-down Pudding. The only problem was, I didn't have half the ingredients, so I drove to the shops, paid to park and fought my way around a packed supermarket. Back home, hot, tired and irritable, I cooked up the pudding. The kitchen looked like a bomb-site and there was a mountain of washing-up. On producing it proudly for the family, my elder son declared that he couldn't eat another thing, my younger son asked didn't I know, he hated pineapple, and my husband said he thought it looked a bit heavy, but he'd have a go. I burst into tears and ended up eating three helpings just to get rid of it.

Later on, feeling fat, I chucked what was left of the whole sorry mess on to the compost heap.

You've probably done something similar to this yourself. I went shopping without a clear meal plan and bought food in the hope that something would come out of it. Not only is this strategy a complete waste of money, it'll also make you fat. It's like buying food to have 'in case someone pops in' (they never do). Unless you're the sort of person who can throw food out without a twinge of conscience, you really must make meal plans in the future. On this diet, you'll know what you're going to buy before each week starts.

4 Lack of willpower

You do have willpower! You want to get back into those jeans or that dress, and you are reading this book. All you have to do now is to keep that goal firmly in your mind.

On this plan I have taken the basic decision-making out of your hands by restricting the range of food available. From there, you can either make up your own meals or you can go with some of my menus. Your willpower will be needed when it comes to raiding the biscuit tin, refusing second helpings and picking at food which you are preparing, but *you have the willpower*. Don't be afraid of hunger while you look forward to your next meal. Don't be tempted to snack. You won't be ill because you already have energy stores there – right on your hips or stomach or thighs! Every time your tummy rumbles and you think you just can't bear it, think of that bit of fat disappearing. If you give in and eat those crisps, the fat will stay exactly where it is. It's as simple as that. Use your willpower and keep your mind focused on those jeans – and how loose they're going to be!

What Will I Be Eating?

You can eat almost anything! Within the rules of the diet, you are free to add up your carbograms to suit yourself. However, I don't like added sugar, I don't allow cakes and biscuits and low-fibre junk food, and I heartily encourage fruits, vegetables and the best wholegrains. You should also choose one or two high-protein foods per day. Proteins assist the absorption of carbohydrates and make their effect longer lasting. Toast on its own has very little satisfaction value and you are hungry again within hours. The addition of an egg, cheese or bacon soon makes for a satisfying meal which will curb hunger for much longer.

In between you can have any amount of vegetables or salads (as long as you count your carbograms). Salad has between 2 and 5cg, a few carrot sticks have 5cg too.

Snacks

You must not eat between meals. This is a rigid rule which works. However much you feel you 'need' something to eat, believe me, if you have excess body fat, you don't. The fat is your fuel. If you keep eating, however low-carbohydrate or low-calorie it is, you are avoiding using that stored fuel. It is also a bad habit to keep putting food into your mouth just because you feel slightly peckish. *Make those food stores work for you.* Every time you go into a fat deficit, those fat stores are being called to action and used up. You are getting slimmer!

Try to eat everything you want in your main meal. You can have a scoop of ice cream, or an after-dinner chocolate mint, but you can't have them between meals. It seems pedantic I know, but it works. *Keep your food for your three mealtimes.* Then brush your teeth, rinse your mouth and tell yourself the meal is over.

The Rules

If I have learned one thing over the years, it is that whatever diet I devise, I can't please everyone. However, most people ask me to set out their meals for them to take away the stress of decision-making. Maybe you are extremely busy or pressured at work, perhaps you have so many people to cater for that you find planning meals too complicated? I will show you how easy it is to be inventive with the food lists. You can either go with my suggestions or plan your own menus.

It doesn't matter whether you're a gourmet, a vegetarian or a harassed parent, male or female, young or not so young, we all want to get back into those jeans – and stay in them for good! In addition to the food lists, there are four other rules:

1 *No* ready-packaged, supermarket convenience meals because you won't be able to tailor their contents to your requirements.
2 *No* more than 1–2 units of alcohol per day.
3 *As little* added sugar as possible – use sugar-free products wherever you can.
4 *No* diet colas, 'low calorie' yoghurts or desserts, or other artificially calorie-reduced products.

You can choose any vegetables from the long list on pages 121–2. They are not entirely free of carbograms and you must still deduct them from your daily allowance, but you can make your own selection.

Have one day off from the diet every week. This is important because the diet is a strict regime from which you need a break every so often. However, on your free day, resist the temptation to eat as much as you can from all your banned foods! Food is *never* a treat. Don't use it as a reward. It's no reward to put your weight back on again and then feel depressed. Remember: the taste of any food only lasts a couple of minutes. *Looking slim lasts a lifetime. The reward is in how you feel about yourself, and how good you look.*

Carbohydrates

Carbohydrates are your most successful diet foods. They are divided into two groups:

Complex*	Simple**
Bread, flour, wholegrains	Sucrose – fruit and vegetables
Pasta	Lactose – milk, yoghurt, etc.
Rice	Fructose – fruit, honey
Vegetables	Maltose – barley, grains
Pulses – peas, beans, etc.	Glucose – vegetables, fruit, honey

* Complex carbohydrates raise the blood-sugar level slowly. Their energy lasts for several hours and they can be used as a base for many meals. About 1,600–2,000 calories can be stored at any one time.

** Simple carbohydrates raise the blood–sugar level quickly, but energy levels also fall quite quickly.

Proteins

After water, protein is the most plentiful substance in the body and it's absolutely vital that you eat enough of it. Think of the wear and tear of living, and how it takes its toll on you. You have worries, you have stresses, you have relationship problems. Your children may be driving you mad, or perhaps you work in a pressured environment. Because of these problems, your immune system takes a battering and the hormones which affect your metabolism, weight and sexual activity are also undergoing constant repair, maintenance and renewal. Only protein can help to repair the damage that has been caused. Typical signs of protein deficiency are falling-out hair, brittle nails and rough skin. You may also suffer from tiredness, anaemia and depression.

Types of protein

There are two types of protein – complete and incomplete. To be complete, a protein has to have eight amino acids, which are classed as essential. They cannot be made by the body and have to be eaten in our food. The best sources of complete proteins come from the following:

- fish
- meat
- eggs
- milk
- dairy products

Some plant proteins are high in quality protein, although they can never be as good as animal proteins. These include:

- soya beans
- brewer's yeast

- nuts
- seeds
- wheat germ

If you exist on a diet that is made up entirely of plant proteins, you will risk protein deficiency. If possible, always try to include at least one complete protein in a meal – cheese, or an egg or milk for example – in order to benefit from maximum good health.

Too much protein

Despite what I've said about how essential it is to eat enough protein, your body doesn't need it in huge quantities. As a rough guide, you need about three-quarters to one gram per kilo of your body weight every day. One example of this amount of protein is that the average person weighing 64 kilos (10 stone) would require just 48–64g of protein per day which can be found in one chicken breast and 568ml (one pint) of milk.

Too much protein is counter-productive because it can't be stored in your body. Excess protein also makes your urine acidic, which leads to a loss of calcium, and most Westerners eat far more protein than they actually need. As a guide, if you're consuming meat, 568ml (one pint) of milk, a cheese sandwhich and an egg breakfast every day, then you are eating too much protein – and far too much saturated fat!

On the other hand, if you are trying to lose weight, it's all too easy to eat too little protein. Living off salads, fruit and vegetables, with just the odd piece of bread or slice of ham, will definitely not give you enough protein and, in time, you'll feel pretty awful. Whether you are studying, working, managing a family or whatever, few of us lead lives that allow us the leisure to feel washed-out half the time – and you'll also look so bad!

How Much Protein Do You Need?

To work out your weight in kilos divide your weight in pounds by 2.2, e.g. 11st 2lb equals 70.9kg. Then multiply 70.9kg by 0.75, which equals 53.18. Therefore if you weighed 70.9kg, you would need 53g of protein a day.

If you are particularly active or sporty, or if you are recovering from an illness, or you are pregnant, increase this to 1g a day per kilo of your body weight. You'll find out exactly how many grams of protein are contained in foods by studying food labels. For example, 568ml (one pint) of milk equals 3.2g protein, 125g (about 5oz) spaghetti equals 10.8g protein.

Fats

You can always tell a person who is obsessed about cutting out fat in their diet because their skin looks dry and flaky. And, as I've already explained, one of the reasons why you may occasionally go berserk and eat everything in sight is because you're eating too little fat (see pages 13–14 and 21–3). It's important to be careful about saturated fats, though, and good as it is, your intake of animal produce *must* be monitored for the sake of your heart. Choose lean meat, don't eat fat or crackling and drink skimmed milk wherever possible. In the weight war, even the so-called 'good' sources of fats, such as those found in nuts, seeds, olive oil and fish, can make you fat if you have too much of them. However, oils found in these foods are brilliant for your health and looks.

For this diet, I have included a special cake recipe (see page 132), which includes lots of lovely seeds and dried fruits. This will be a real treat and it will help give you the fats you need.

Once you start eating the right amounts of fats you should find that your food cravings vanish and this will be a major breakthrough in the weight war.

A word of warning about 'fat-reduced' and 'fat-less' claims: the general move in the food industry to reduce fat content is undoubtedly good. The problem comes, though, when people eat fat-reduced food when they might otherwise have eaten nothing at all – or too much of it, as they think they have more leeway. I have actually heard a fellow shopper saying she didn't want any crisps, then changing her mind when a certain label caught her eye. 'Oh, I could have these low-fat ones, instead,' she said. Instead of what? Instead of not having anything at all?

Don't be fooled: even healthy food can contain a lot of calories. If you're going to win the weight war, you must take note of calories from *all* sources.

Sugar

For years, my job as a diet counsellor has been to keep beautiful women slim in the face of gruelling schedules and constant entertaining. I devise personal diets for them and my low-sugar or sugar-free diet has always been one of the most popular and successful.

On *The New Get Back Into Your Jeans Diet* your added sugar intake must be cut. Natural sugars are already found in many foods, such as milk and vegetables, and we could not function well without them, but added sugar is totally unnecessary for your body. You should cut it out altogether.

On average, each person in Britain buys and eats 40 kilos of sugar every year. Even if you think you don't eat a lot yourself, you may not have a choice. Half the sugar you eat is 'hidden' – added in by some food manufacturers to enhance flavour. This all adds up to the obesity and weight troubles of the nation, and, in my opinion, it is a scandal that is not taken seriously enough. Sugar rots your teeth and adds 'empty' calories to your intake – ones you can't use. There are just three main foods with empty calories: sugar, lard and alcohol. Watch out for them!

Twenty years ago I used to diet like a maniac. I was always hungry, but I was also slim. I was constantly tired and washed-out – but I was slim. It all seemed worth it, but I didn't count sugar as one of the main reasons why I felt so exhausted – instead of eating sensibly I was using it for a boost. My diet biscuits couldn't be so bad, I thought, that low-calorie chocolate bar was fine, and I could fill up the rest of the day on fruit. However, I slept badly and, quite frankly, was a different woman. I decided to cut out added sugar to keep my son company when he was suddenly diagnosed as being a diabetic, and I have never looked back. Today, without the aid of supplements or tablets of any kind, I have the energy and vitality to work a sixteen-hour day, and my figure is better than it was when I was twenty-five. Finding sugar-free alternatives is easy, and you can lose your sweet tooth altogether, especially if you keep up your carbohydrates.

There are two types of sugars: *extrinsic*, which means sugars that are not naturally present in food as they have been added, and *intrinsic* sugars, which are part of the food. Examples of these are as follows:

Intrinsic (no restriction)	Extrinsic (limit to 60g a day)
Milk	Table sugar
Starches	Jams
Fruit	Biscuits
Vegetables	Cakes
	Sweets and chocolate

How much sugar do I need?

The World Health Organization recommends a daily intake of added sugar to be no higher than 60g a day (or 10 per cent of your total calories). So, on a 1,500 calorie-a-day diet, you should eat no more than 150 calories of sugar.

Foods with 'hidden' sugar

Here are some examples of typical foods with added sugar before they even get to you!

Coco Pops (per 30g serving)	12.0g sugar
1 slice chocolate Swiss roll	20.5g
Seafood sauce (per 100ml)	14.6g
Chicken vindaloo (340g)	13.9g
Ready-made coleslaw (100g)	5.8g
Cheese and pickle sandwich	12.5g
Can cream of tomato soup (290g)	15.6g
Nutri-grain 98 per cent fat-free	12.0g

As a comparison, here are some ways of cutting sugar:

Shredded Wheat (30g)	0.1g sugar
Profiterole (with cream and small chocolate topping!)	3.9g
Home-made mayonnaise (1dsp)	1.3g
Tandoori breast of chicken	3.0g
Home-made coleslaw (100g)	1.2g
Roast beef or chicken sandwich	1.2g
Bowl fresh lentil soup	1.7g
Go-Ahead Chocolina (each)	3.4g

Making the Right Choices

Always study food labels as these give precise information about carbohydrate and sugar contents, as well as other nutritional values (see also page 47). The big retail chains have recently introduced new labelling which shows at a glance into which category a product falls:

Sugar-free *contains no added or natural sugars*
No added sugar *no sugars added from any source*
Low-sugar *less than 5g of sugar including those naturally present*
Reduced sugar *at least 25 per cent less sugar than the standard product – but beware, as the original product may have had a lot of sugar in it in the first place!*

It is easy to make the right food choices. *Take control of your diet. Don't let anyone else load you with unwanted calories.* The first two categories are really the ones to look out for – but remember, don't buy or eat something just because it's low in sugar or sugar-free: keep track of the calories as well.

Your CarboRange

Your limit on carbohydrates in this diet is 120–150g – known as your CarboRange. By setting a limit on carbohydrates, you begin to value them. You choose items you really want rather than squandering everything on naan bread or a can of something fizzy to drink.

Revising Carbograms Downwards – Will It Mean More Weight Loss?

As you lose weight, you might reach the depressing 'plateau' stage where your weight loss sticks and you stay the same weight for weeks. When this happens to clients of mine they get extremely fed up that although they are sticking to their diet rigidly, nothing happens. The temptation to throw in the towel and eat a massive takeaway is almost irresistible!

In almost all cases, they are getting slack about either portion sizes or nibbles. It feels like nothing to have a bite out of someone's sandwich or the odd fruit pastille. Well, a recent experiment I conducted revealed that one client's two pastilles a day habit actually added up to 560 calories a week – more than a roast chicken dinner. Yes, two stupid sweets were actually an entire *extra meal*. It seems mean to deny someone their two sweets and in the normal course of events it wouldn't matter a bit, but if you are trying to lose weight you have to take notice of these things.

I think it is better to reduce portion sizes generally, which will reduce overall calories. You need energy for exercise, and carbohydrates are your energy. It is better to work off the calories – don't groan – with a 40-minute walk, 20 minutes swimming or just cleaning the car with extra vigour instead of taking it to the car wash. These activities will get that weight moving again, I promise.

Reading Food Labels

Counting carbograms and finding out how much sugar is in your food is not as hard, time-consuming or as fiddly as you may think. Yes, at first it takes a bit of concentration and effort, but soon you will be able to glance at a label and know instantly whether it is the right food for you. Knowledge is power: I used to find I had been eating some things for years without realizing just how bad they were for me!

As I've already explained, the two most important pieces of information for following *The New Get Back Into Your Jeans Diet* are carbohydrate and sugar content. Here is an example of a typical food label from a breakfast cereal:

Nutrition Information

Typical values	Per 100g	Per 30g serving
Energy	387kcal	116kcal
Protein	6.5g	2.0g
Carbohydrates	85.5g	26.0g
(of which sugars)	49.0g	14.7g
Fat	1.0g	0.3g
(of which saturates)	0.2g	0.06g
Fibre	3.0g	0.9g
Sodium	trace	trace

There are three very important pieces of information contained here. First, the fat content is low and the *saturated* fat content is extremely low at only 0.06g per 30g – the size of a typical bowlful of this particular cereal. However, this information can be slightly misleading when it is used by slimmers on their weight-loss plans. Note that the added sugar content is 14.7g per serving, nearly *three times* the sugar content of many sugar-free cereals. As you will be counting carbohydrates on this diet, the information that this cereal contains 26g of carbohydrates is also useful.

It's worth mentioning too that the lower-fat content of this particular cereal does not mean it is low-calorie. It has sixteen calories *more* per bowlful than sugar-free cereals. It may seem a bother to read labels and count calories, but you won't mind when you see your thighs getting slimmer and your bottom becoming smaller – and when you get back into those jeans that you've always dreamed of wearing again!

Vitamins

What do they do?

Vitamin requirements vary according to lifestyle and age, but we all need the right balance of vitamins to feel well and to function properly. For example, lack of iron makes you feel tired and breathless, while lack of vitamin C can lead to aching joints and sore gums. Children need more vitamins than adults simply because they are still growing and developing, but it is also possible to overdo it. Excess vitamins and minerals can cause their own problems, and for further details you should consult a good natural health reference book. But this shouldn't be a reason not to take sensible doses of supplements when you are eating a good diet.

What vitamins can't do is give you energy. Many people feel that a spell of tiredness and stress, and especially feelings of weakness and lethargy, can be overcome by popping mega-doses of pills. It doesn't work like this! Vitamins do *not* give you energy – they don't have any calories! Only calories can give you energy and, as you have already learned, calories come from food. You see, you do need the right ones!

Ideally, you should gain all the vitamins and minerals that you need from your food. But good reasons to take extra vitamins may be in times of great stress, illness, pregnancy or lack of appetite, when nutrients could be missing from your diet, or your condition may be draining you of nutrients. *Never use pills as a substitute for food, but as a supplement.*

Here is your guide to the essential vitamins, where to find them, how much you need – and how much is too much! If in any doubt as to your own needs or restrictions, consult your doctor.

The Essential Vitamins

Vitamin	Where Found	Symptoms of Deficiency	Symptoms of Excess	Daily Requirements
Vitamin A	Cheese Kidneys Eggs Butter Fish oils Apricots Peppers Carrots	Fragile bones Loss of appetite Sight problems	Hair loss Headache Vomiting Defects in new babies	50g carrots or a slice liver
Vitamin B1	Potatoes Kidneys Beans Peas Cereals	Swelling limbs Confusion Muscle weakness Loss of sensation	None known	4 tbsp rice or 6 slices wholemeal bread
Vitamin B2	Chicken Fish Meat Milk Eggs Cereals	Cracked lips Bloodshot eyes Skin problems	None known	1 bowl cereal
Vitamin B6	Cereals Nuts Bananas Yeast Eggs Soya beans	Deficiency is rare	Nerve damage to hands and feet	1 bowl cereal or 1 portion fish
Vitamin B12	Meat Chicken Dairy products Fish	Tiredness Pins and needles	None known	1 glass milk or 1 portion fish

Vitamin	Where Found	Symptoms of Deficiency	Symptoms of Excess	Daily Requirements
Niacin	Peas Beans Sweetcorn Nuts Cereals Potatoes Meat	Tiredness Skin rashes Diarrhoea Depression	High doses could result in flushed skin	1 piece fish, meat or chicken
Folic Acid	Spinach Broccoli Cereals Watercress Bread	Wasting of the gut because nutrients cannot be properly absorbed	None known	2 portions vegetables or 4 glasses orange juice
Vitamin C	Potatoes Apples Citrus fruits Vegetables	Aching joints Fatigue Sore gums Bone pain Loss of appetite Scaly skin	Excess is mostly excreted in urine and mega-doses can cause disturbed sleep	1 orange or potato
Vitamin E	Wheatgerm Nuts Seeds Vegetable oils Margarines Fish oils	Deficiency is rare	None known	30g nuts

Minerals

We all need a wide range of minerals to maintain health and for the following bodily functions:

- strong bones and teeth
- a healthy immune system
- to enable vitamins to work

The Essential Minerals

Minerals	Where Found	Symptoms of Deficiency	Symptoms of Excess	Daily Requirements
Calcium	Milk and other dairy products Sardines Sesame seeds Green leafy vegetables	Muscle weakness Back pain Soft and brittle bones	Loss of appetite Vomiting Constipation	800–1000mg
Magnesium	Wheatgerm Beans Peas Nuts Sesame seeds Figs	Tiredness Weakness Cramps Chocolate cravings	None known	300mg
Potassium	Avocados Bananas Fresh and dried fruits Beans Peas Mushrooms Tomatoes	Extreme thirst Weakness Tiredness	None known	3.5g
Sodium	Tinned anchovies Table salt Marmite	Dehydration Cramps Low blood pressure	High blood pressure	1600mg

Minerals	Where Found	Symptoms of Deficiency	Symptoms of Excess	Daily Requirements
Iron	Egg yolks Sardines Dark green vegetables Offal Beef	Breathlessness Tiredness	Excess rare	8.7mg (men) 14.8mg (women)
Selenium	Brazil nuts Meat and fish Avocados Lentils	Deficiency is rare	Toxic in excess, it causes foul breath and body odour. Excess would be above 450mcg/day	50–75mcg

Your Basic Foods

The basic foods on this diet are simple, because the foods with the lowest carbograms – and therefore the ones you can eat the most of – are also low in added sugar and fat. Your foods must be fresh.

1. You should eat a diet which contains 120–150cg a day and this should include four pieces of fresh fruit or their equivalent per day.
2. A quarter litre skimmed (15cg) or soya milk (2.3cg) per day – the carbograms are not included in your basic allowance and you will not have to include them – they are extra.
3. Seven grams of butter per day. Butter contains only a trace of carbohydrates.
4. Up to three portions of high-protein food a day.

'Can I Just Ask You Something?'

Every day my telephone rings and there is a new client on the other end who has just embarked on the first week of her diet. You may have some (or all) of the same queries, so it's best to deal with them before you get going. These are based on real people's questions.

I don't understand – it sounds like I can have a massive steak and vegetables and still have enough carbograms for pudding, but you don't agree with this. Surely if I keep within my carbogram budget, I could eat nothing but cakes and sweets all day, if that is what I want?

You would think that, wouldn't you? But it doesn't work like that. You have to eat at least two protein portions a day, something like salmon or chicken, and you aren't likely to eat them just on their own. You must also have a serving of cereal with milk. I have insisted on this because you need the fibre, iron, calcium and all the other good things in this meal. So you are going to be left with too few carbograms to start indulging in slices of pie and choc ices.

Remember why you are doing this. Losing weight is one thing, but the purpose of this diet is its entire effect. It is no good being slimmer if your face is covered in spots. It is no good weighing less if your hair is dull and coarse. This is what you will look like if you start living off sweets and cakes. *The New Get Back Into Your Jeans Diet* is healthy, wholesome and, ultimately, a beauty diet as well as an energy diet and a weight-loss or a weight-maintenance diet. Eating cakes and sweets is not really part of a grown woman's diet, except for special occasions or when someone has gone to the trouble of making you something and you simply can't get out of eating it. This is why I have given you a list (see page 76) showing you the carbogram values of some sweets and puddings. I don't recommend you blow your carbogram budget on them more than once a month, if that.

You allow 120–150 carbograms a day. How do I know how many I need?
It doesn't matter. This is a range within which you should eat. What I am saying is that if the limit was rigid, say 120cg a day, and the meal you wanted was 124cg, you would be fretting over how to cut down by four carbograms when it really is neither here nor there. If you want to lose weight a little faster, go for the lower limit. If you prefer higher-carbohydrate meals, you have those 50cg to use on a jacket potato, possibly, or some extra rice with your curry. You might also be housebound or disabled or getting over surgery and therefore less active, in which case the 120cg limit is better for you.

Do I really have to keep weighing everything? It seems such a chore and I can't really be bothered.
You don't have to do anything. And you don't have to go on this diet. No one is telling you to do anything against your will, but if you're determined to succeed and to get back into those jeans, then you need to take some steps in the right direction. That means weighing food, because it was by *not* weighing it and by guessing portions that you gained weight in the first place. It was by not being bothered and eating whatever took your fancy that you gained weight. I'm not suggesting there's

anything wrong with eating whatever you fancy if you're happy, but if you're reading this book you're probably not and it's resulted in a figure that you don't want. So make the effort. It doesn't go on for ever because you'll soon get to know what 50g of cereal looks like and how heavy a serving of pasta is without getting out the scales. Take heart: weighing takes just a few seconds, but being slim and getting back into those clothes is a pleasure which is reinforced every time you look in the mirror.

The fruit allowance is rather small. I love fruit and eat it by the barrowful. Why can't I have more?

Eating fruit 'by the barrowful' is lovely and healthy, but unfortunately it also contains calories just like anything else! Remember, the idea of this diet is to encourage a more balanced view of food and constant snacking is probably a problem for you. Over the next month you should try to retrain yourself through restriction, and then you can go back to your barrowfuls of fruit if you still want to – but I'll bet you're unlikely to want to, and will have learned to keep an eye out for those calories.

Am I allowed to drink alcohol on this diet?

Yes, but look at the carbograms. Your limit is one or two alcoholic drinks per day. On the suggested menus I have given a few drinks here and there, but feel free to make up your own carbogram menus and choose your own drinks to fit in with your allowance.

You don't allow diet colas on this diet, or diet drinks in general. I find them useful to curb my hunger pangs and they have no calories. Why can't I have them?

If you're hungry, your body needs *food*. Remember what I said about cravings and your body trying to talk to you? Hunger is a message. But I do believe for good weight maintenance that you should stick to mealtimes and scheduled food breaks. After you've retrained yourself, the hunger pangs will stop, but in the meantime, don't dampen them with fizzy drinks; have pure water instead. Most diet drinks contain caffeine, which is addictive and bad for you, and they also contain high levels of artificial sweeteners which only encourage your sweet tooth. Stay away from them. Wait for your meal, drink water, and your food will taste all the better because you have looked forward to it.

Why no diet yoghurts or desserts?
Most of them still contain sugar or other additives which can cause bloating and flatulence. They are also pumped full of air so you seem to be getting more than there really is, and at the end of the day they can be unsatisfying. It is far better to have pure, unadulterated live yoghurt with fresh or dried fruit to give you that bit of sweetness which you are used to after a meal.

I just want to get my stomach smaller – the rest of me is fine. How can this diet help me?
You need to read my book, *5 Days to a Flatter Stomach* (Boxtree), which has a similar diet but concentrates on the other causes of a big stomach, such as bloating. For example, you're allowed fruit, but only in the evenings. You're allowed vegetables, but not pulses, broccoli or sprouts. And you can only eat white bread. That diet will also help you because its main theme is frequent eating and this has been proved to be an important factor in getting your stomach flat.

Will this diet help me to reduce fat on my thighs?
The whole plan, including the exercise, will help, yes. No diet can target thighs or any other part of your body, but if you carry your excess fat on your thighs, it's likely that this is where it will go from. I think you'll have spectacular results.

I am semi-disabled and have arthritis in both knees. I can't exercise much, but I am desperate to lose weight as I am 16 stone-plus. Will this diet work for me?

Yes it will – in fact this diet is the most effective for people with low-energy requirements because you don't want to be filling yourself with a lot of high-energy foods if you don't need them. The only specific advice for people with arthritis is to avoid potatoes, peppers, aubergines and tomatoes as they are particularly likely to aggravate inflammatory conditions. But there is still a lot to choose from, and you should get relief from your problems simply by losing some weight.

I lead a hectic life as a community nurse and often have to take meal breaks in my car. How can I possibly fit this diet into my lifestyle?

You still have to eat! I have included 'snacker's' menus which divide up the basic foods for you into five or six small snacks (see pages 82–4). The secret lies in the planning and what you must avoid at all costs is going for hours on end without eating and then having too much in the evening. As long as you plan ahead and prepare food when it's convenient to do so, such as on a Sunday, you should have a fridge stocked and ready for you to devise a week's home-made diet snacks.

I go out to eat a lot as the job I do involves a lot of socializing for business. How can I stick to a diet when I have to eat restaurant food?

There's nothing special about restaurant food! Most menus have plain fish or meat, salads and vegetables, and they're the best to go for. A word of advice: don't go for risottos or pasta dishes when you are out as I have seen the amount of butter and oils that can be poured over them, and ask if the restaurant adds butter to their vegetables before serving. If they do, ask them not to. Ask for sauces to be left off meat or fish, too.

It's bad manners to go without a course when everyone else is having one, so always choose something and then pick at it. If there isn't a fruit option for pudding and everyone is having one, choose anything – it doesn't matter what – and have half of it. It won't break your calorie bank.

I'm not used to this kind of diet and I feel out of control. I'm not sure that I want to be told what to eat.

You have two options: to stay as you are or to go forward. No one is forcing you into either choice, but please understand: you weren't in control before, which is why you have this problem. Your appetite was controlling you. Now you truly are in the driving seat because you are strong enough to resist temptation. The process is a bit hard at first because you are breaking yourself of old habits. But very soon you will have the eating habits of a slim person and you will emerge 'reinvented'.

Your Personal Measurement Record

First of all, you need to know where you're starting from. You should weigh and measure yourself so that you can monitor where the weight is going from, or which bits are being toned up. Write down your current clothes size too. When you have filled in your details, don't check them again for two weeks. In a month's time you will be able to compare your first and last charts, and hopefully you'll have a wonderful surprise!

The reason for measuring the area just underneath the bust-line is because weight is often stored on – and lost from – your back. Therefore, the general bust measurement can be mistaken for breast size when it incorporates your back and weight loss that registers on scales often can't be seen. 'I've lost weight –

but I don't know where from!' is a common cry from my clients. Only by exercising and toning will you be sure that the stubborn areas of fat that stop you from getting back into those jeans are slimmed down.

Keep this record to remind you where you lost the weight.

Personal Measurement Record

Date ....

Weight .... kg

Bust .... cm

Chest (men) .... cm

Under bust (ribcage) .... cm

Waist .... cm

Pelvis (hip bones) .... cm

Hips .... cm

Top of the thigh .... cm

Above the knee .... cm

Dress size ....

After Two Weeks

Weight .... kg

Bust .... cm

Chest (men) .... cm

Under bust (ribcage) .... cm

Waist .... cm

Pelvis (hip bones) .... cm

Hips .... cm

Top of the thigh .... cm

Above the knee .... cm

Dress size ....

At the End of the Month

Weight .... kg

Bust .... cm

Chest (men) .... cm

Under bust (ribcage) .... cm

Waist .... cm

Pelvis (hip bones) .... cm

Hips .... cm

Top of the thigh .... cm

Above the knee .... cm

Dress size ....

Menus For A Month

The idea is that you take control from here and make up your own menus for the rest of your life. But to get you started, and to a certain extent to get you re-programmed to counting carbohydrates, I have given you some ideas here. You don't have to follow these menus to the letter, but you will start to lose weight with them as they are carefully checked for carbograms. I have also given you some other options depending on the sort of person you are: you might love or loathe cooking; you might eat on the run or be housebound. I hope I have something for everyone but if not, it is easy to write it all down and keep your own food record.

- Drink plain water with your meals.
- No more than two alcoholic drinks per day.
- Keep your food diary.
- Check your carbograms all the time until you get used to them. Remember you are allowed 120–150cg per day (men or very tall women should take the higher limit). This means do not go below 120cg and not above 150cg.

Keeping A Food Diary

Whenever a new client comes to me, their first task is to keep a food diary for a week, which I can then analyse. They mustn't try to impress me or to hide anything, and they write down everything that passes their lips during those seven days, even if it is a lick of the spoon while making a cake. This gives me an idea of their eating habits as well as what they are actually eating. Then, when I have given them their personal diet, they continue to keep a record, and you will be keeping the same sort of diary for yourself.

It may seem tedious, but after a month the diary isn't necessary. You can go back to it whenever problems arise because it is a good way to spot extra carbograms. People don't think that the extra bite of carrot makes any difference, and in a way it doesn't, but add up all the bites and they can easily amount to an extra 20g of carbohydrate in a day – especially if sugar was involved. You won't become a carbogram fanatic, just develop a sixth sense about your food and care about your body. You can still enjoy food and have tasty meals as long as you monitor yourself and are active. This is what people mean when they say 'I'm careful'.

Why Bother?

You try to watch your eating for three reasons:

1 You can see the carbograms you consume through tasting, nibbling and picking at food.
2 You realize the carbogram content of 'good' foods such as salads, fruit and vegetables, which can still mount up.
3 It allows you to be in control and to decide just how you want to distribute your carbograms during each day. This means that you can save carbograms for special occasions and still not gain weight.

How To Keep The Diary

Leave your diary in the kitchen, car or office desk – wherever it will be most handy for you. I have written some sample pages (see pages 67–9) and you simply deduct carbograms as you go along. Start with the foods you know you are going to have, such as your milk allowance, cereal and so on, then you'll know how many carbograms you have left for the rest of the day.

Deducting carbograms is a more efficient and successful way of monitoring your food intake than adding them up. You only have to keep this diary for the next month, so stick with it! You're going to be lighter, more shapely and slimmer – *and* you're going to get back into those jeans!

Your Daily Record

Keeping a Daily Carbogram Record is incredibly easy and convenient. Nobody eats all the food in the world and most of us have a very limited range of meals. Whether this is a good thing or not, it is a fact of life. For example, my own daily diet revolves around porridge, salads, tuna fish, cheese, fruit and potatoes. I eat other meals obviously, but not that often, just as you probably stick to the same meals – you head for the same sandwiches, grab the same yoghurt or packet of crisps at the same time of day, day in and day out. We're all creatures of habit. Habit is probably what made you gain weight in the first place, because you simply couldn't put in the mental effort and energy to find new habits. It's not a crime, but it *is* laziness. Changing your diet means wrenching yourself 360 degrees to head the other way, but once you get the idea, you can have a favourite meal every day if it makes things easier for you. A daily record is a sensible way to get started as it helps you to stay within your CarboRange. You can find a list of foods with their carbogram values in the Food File section but here are some examples to give you an idea of how things work:

Food eaten:	Starting cg allowance. 150 (milk included)
Less a 30cg breakfast	120
Less 1 piece fruit, 10cg	110
Less a 10cg salad lunch	100
Less a 60cg jacket potato dinner	40
Less 3-fruit salad, 1 glass wine, 31cg	9
Less a soya yoghurt as snack, 5cg	4

You have successfully gone 4cg under your daily CarboRange

Other ways of doing it:

Example A
You like a good breakfast and lunch, but don't eat much in the evening.

Breakfast:	**30cg range** Bacon, eggs, tomatoes Porridge with milk
Lunch:	**90cg range** Jacket potato with tuna Fruit salad
Dinner:	**You have 30cg remaining** Roast chicken with 3 vegetables 1 piece fruit
Total:	**150 carbograms**

Example B

You are going out for dinner tonight and want to save some carbograms for dessert.

Breakfast:	**20cg**
	Mixed fruit salad
	2-egg omelette
Lunch:	**20cg**
	Avocado with prawns *or* ham salad
	Apple
Dinner:	**110cg remaining for this meal**
	2 glasses wine
	Spaghetti Bolognese
	Ice cream dessert
	Coffee with 2 chocolates
Total:	**150 carbograms**

Example C

You are travelling today and it is going to be difficult to have a proper meal.

Breakfast:	**30cg**
	Cereal with milk
	Grapefruit segments
Snack lunch:	**35cg**
	Sandwich
Snack:	**30cg**
	Banana
	Apple
Light meal:	**20cg**
	Tuna salad
	Few grapes or a satsuma

Light meal:	**55cg**
	Bagel with cream cheese
	Fruit
Total:	**10cg over your CarboRange for this day**

Protein Foods

Choose one from this list for every meal to a maximum of three portions a day. You may have two portions in one meal, eggs and bacon for example, but try not to exceed three portions a day. You need protein with carbohydrate to help absorption.

- 1 tbsp nuts
- 3 slices chicken
- small skinless chicken breast
- 3 slices roast beef, pork, lamb, etc.
- 1 steak, pork or lamb chop
- 150g Quorn or tofu
- pouch or half a tin tuna fish
- fillet any white fish
- 1–3 eggs
- 3 tbsp prawns or crabmeat
- 3 slices smoked salmon
- small stick hard cheese (not cottage)
- small tub or 3 tbsp cottage cheese – 3cg
- tin sardines
- portion smoked mackerel
- medium serving liver
- 3 rashers lean bacon
- 3 slices lean ham
- 2 slices hard cheese

A Day Of Rest?

Having a diet break is an interesting point. It depends on whether you see this as a lifestyle diet or a 'results' diet and I'll explain the difference. Bodybuilders go on results diets. So do sportspeople. They follow a rigid regime for the sole purpose of performing better, reducing body fat, increasing muscle, or whatever, and they build days off into their schedule. A bodybuilder will have a deliberate off-season when he expects to gain 5 kilos, then he would diet quite rigorously to get to peak condition for competition, losing that weight quite deliberately. A footballer has several weeks off season when he would take little exercise, eat quite normally and expect to gain weight. During the season he would eat according to a nutritionist's advice and get lean again. Results diets are good for weddings and holidays and other special occasions, but like the previous examples they assume that you are in quite good condition before you start. All you are losing is maybe 5 kilos and getting back to where you were before. People who do results dieting can be strict for six days and enjoy a pudding and a few glasses of wine on the seventh. But results diets are hopeless for self-confessed gluttons, the severely overweight or people with a genuinely unhealthy approach to their diet because these types of diets assume a measure of self-control and discipline which this category is unlikely to have.

People with bad habits need lifestyle diets like this one. It is a total change in attitude and a way of re-training your habits. I personally feel that a day off a lifestyle diet is the beginning of the slow slide back to what you were doing before. It is like allowing an alcoholic one drink or an ex-smoker a cigarette. Sometimes you just have to accept that you have a problem with food and you must give up some things for good. Therefore I don't recommend that you have a day off, but if you are a true 'results' dieter, I leave it to your discretion.

THE DIET

Choose between 120–150cg units. You may either follow the recommended menus on pages 76–89 or choose your meals from these lists. Meals should *only* use these recommended foods.

TO DRINK

Plain water – at least 8 glasses every day

Fruit teas

Herbal teas

Standard tea

Decaffeinated coffee – can be drunk freely

Coffee – two cups a day

Alcohol – 2 glasses a day maximum

BREAKFASTS

0–5cg

Smoked haddock and poached egg

Scrambled eggs with milk

3 rashers bacon, 1 egg, poached or scrambled

3 rashers bacon, tomatoes and mushrooms

Smoked salmon and scrambled egg

2- or 3-egg omelette

20cg

2 slices of toast, butter and boiled egg

Porridge made with water

1 slice of toast, butter, 2 tsp marmalade

1 slice of toast with grilled cheese

Egg on toast

30cg

Serving of any cereal from list, with average serving of milk

Mixed 3-fruit salad

35cg

2 slices of toast with butter and a boiled or scrambled egg
2 tbsp baked beans on 1 slice toast
Banana and plain yoghurt
2 slices of cheese on 2 slices of toast
2 scrambled eggs on 2 slices of toast
Bacon sandwich

45cg

2 slices of toast, butter, 2 tsp marmalade
Bagel with cream cheese and/or smoked salmon
Large fruit compote – prunes, apricots, sultanas, figs
Cereal topped with 1 dsp fruit compote and milk
Cereal with fruit compote and 1 dsp yoghurt
Milk, banana, yoghurt and other fruit as a 'smoothie'

LIGHT MEALS OR LUNCHES
Salads
2cg

Any amount of salad leaves such as lettuce, cucumber, rocket,
watercress, lamb's lettuce, and radishes, parsley, asparagus spears
with 1 dsp French dressing or 1 tsp mayonnaise

10cg

Mixed salad. Any standard mixed salad including tomatoes,
grated beetroot, grated carrot, coloured peppers, radishes,
onions, sweetcorn
Any mixed salad with a serving of ham, cheese, chicken, tuna, etc.
½ avocado and bacon with green salad
Any mixed salad with your daily allowance of nuts or toasted
pine nuts
Green salad with 2 tbsp peas
½ avocado with smoked salmon, prawns or bacon bits,
served on green salad

25cg
Soup and roll
Small roll filled with salad, ham, cheese, chicken, tuna, etc.
4 cream crackers and cheese
4 Ryvitas and cheese, cottage cheese or tuna
Thin slice quiche and salad

35cg
All sandwiches (2 slices bread)
with ham, chicken, cheese or salad filling
2 tbsp baked beans on 1 slice of toast
Winter salad – grated raw red and white cabbage, carrot, onion,
½ an apple, grated and tossed in lemon, walnuts and a
sprinkling sultanas (about one dessertspoon)

50cg
Baguette, bagel, croissant, pitta bread with filling and/or salad
Medium slice quiche with salad
Medium slice pizza with salad

60cg
Jacket potatoes:
with cheese or cottage cheese
with tuna
with ham
with any meat and vegetables, using a smaller potato
with butter from allowance
with 1 tbsp sour cream and chive dressing
salad with any of the above

MAIN MEALS
Starters
(either eating out, as an appetizer at home or
as a light evening meal)

10cg
Corn on the cob
Slice of melon
Slice melon with raspberries
Bowl asparagus, watercress, carrot soup, etc. (see label for
carbohydrate values per serving – soups with potatoes or flour
thickening will have higher carbohydrates)
Grapefruit segments
Prawns in dressing with salad
Mussels
Smoked salmon, ½ slice bread
Smoked mackerel, salad, ½ slice bread

20cg
All the following meals can be served with two or three
vegetables, including:
asparagus
cabbage
sprouts
swede
carrot and swede
turnip
kale
parsnip
peas
sweetcorn
broccoli
cauliflower
any other vegetables to suit

Roast meat from allowance
Portion 'shepherd's type' pie with parsnip mash instead of
potato mash on top
Pork or lamb chop with gravy

Meat, poultry or seafood curry with light sauce
Cod or haddock in white/parsley sauce
Chicken stir-fry with mixed vegetables, soy sauce
Beef or prawn stir-fry
Fillet steak with salad, mushrooms, peas
Salmon fillet, grilled or pan-fried
Cod or haddock, plain grilled or oven-baked
2-egg omelette

35cg
Home-made fresh vegetable soup (including potatoes)
Serve these meals with salad *or* 2–3 vegetables:
Small serving lasagne
Small portion shepherd's pie
Portion chilli con carne with 2 dsp rice (½ portion)
Salade Niçoise

50cg
All the meals above, with the addition of 2 small boiled potatoes
or 2 spoonfuls mashed potato.

80cg
Any curry with 3–4 tbsp rice
Chilli con carne with rice
Spaghetti Bolognese with portion pasta
Pasta shapes with vegetable sauce
Pasta shapes with smoked salmon and crème fraîche
Poached cod in caper sauce with lime rice
Pasta twists with pesto and nut dressing
Lasagne Verde
Kedgeree

EXTRA PORTIONS
All 60cg
Standard portion of restaurant chips
Portion of rice 4 tbsp
Portion of pasta
Jacket potato
4–5 tbsp couscous

PUDDINGS AND DESSERTS
20cg
Mixed fresh fruit salad. This might be made with 3–4 fruits,
but assume a 3 tbsp serving
One low-fat fruit yoghurt
½ banana and 3 tbsp custard
Small pot plain 'bio' yoghurt (or 3 tbsp)
2 scoops ice cream

30cg
3 tbsp stewed fruit with sugar
Small slice cheesecake
Small slice fruit pie

EXTRAS
1 tsp sugar (in tea, coffee, etc.) 5cg
Packet sugar (in coffee shops) 7cg
1 after-dinner mint 6cg

Standard Menus

These daily menus should suit you if you prefer having your
meals set out for you. Each menu is within your daily Carbo-
Range of 120–150 units (or very slightly above), but you should

not mix and match – each day is carefully balanced and all the meals for that day should be taken. However you can choose any day that you want, and you can have the same day up to three times a week (but no more than this).

─────── Day 1 ───────

BREAKFAST
Cereal and milk
Glass of orange juice

MID-MORNING
Mixed salad and dressing

LUNCH
Any sandwich
Apple

MAIN MEAL
Chicken stir-fry
2 pieces fruit

─────── Day 2 ───────

BREAKFAST
1 egg and 2 slices of toast
½ grapefruit

MID-MORNING
Banana and a drink

LUNCH
Salad with cheese or meat
Small bunch grapes

MAIN MEAL
Portion of lasagne with salad
Mango and pineapple salad
Glass of wine
After-dinner mint

─────── Day 3 ───────

BREAKFAST
Portion of muesli with milk
Sliced apple

MID-MORNING
Piece of fruit

LUNCH
4 crispbreads with cottage cheese
Fruit

MAIN MEAL
Jacket potato, barbecued or roast
    chicken
Piece of fruit

─────── Day 4 ───────

BREAKFAST
2 slices of toast and marmalade

MID-MORNING
Apple

LUNCH
Any sandwich
Banana

MAIN MEAL
Lamb chop, 3 vegetables
Grape and melon salad

Day 5

BREAKFAST
Porridge with milk
1 slice of toast with butter

MID-MORNING
Piece of fruit

LUNCH
Cottage cheese and fruit platter
(3 fruits)

MAIN MEAL
Salmon fillet with 3 vegetables
and a portion of new potatoes
Glass of wine
2 after-dinner mints

Day 6

BREAKFAST
3-fruit mixed salad, including
banana

MID-MORNING
2 Ryvitas with a slice of cheese

LUNCH
Ham or tuna salad with dressing

MAIN MEAL
2 tbsp baked beans on 2 slices of
toast
Sliced strawberries with crème or
fromage frais *or* sliced mango

Day 7

BREAKFAST
2 scrambled eggs, 2 slices of toast
Apple

LUNCH
½ avocado filled with prawns,
salad

MAIN MEAL
Jacket potato with large,
colourful mixed salad
3-fruit salad

Vegetarian Menus

—————— Day 1 ——————

BREAKFAST
Cereal and milk

MID-MORNING
Apple

LUNCH
Salad sandwich
Grapes

MAIN MEAL
Szechuan pepper and tofu stir-fry
2 pieces fruit

—————— Day 2 ——————

BREAKFAST
Cereal and milk or soya milk

MID-MORNING
Apple

LUNCH
Tuna baguette with salad

MAIN MEAL
Avocado and pine nut salad
3-fruit salad

—————— Day 3 ——————

BREAKFAST
2 fruits with sultanas and
    yoghurt

MID-MORNING
Small roll and butter

LUNCH
Any mixed salad
Bunch grapes

MAIN MEAL
Pasta twists with pesto and nut
    dressing

—————— Day 4 ——————

BREAKFAST
Cereal and milk, sultanas

MID-MORNING
Apple

LUNCH
Any sandwich
Orange

MAIN MEAL
Omelette with salad
Glass of wine

Day 5

BREAKFAST
Porridge made with water, 1 tsp
  honey

MID-MORNING
Apple

LUNCH
Cottage cheese on 4 crispbreads

MAIN MEAL
Lasagne Verde and salad
2 fruits

Day 6

BREAKFAST
Cereal and soya milk
Glass of orange juice

MID-MORNING
Carrot and celery sticks with tub
  of cottage cheese

LUNCH
Mixed fruit and banana salad

MAIN MEAL
Red bean and tomato curry
or baked beans on 2 slices of
  toast

Day 7

BREAKFAST
2 Weetabix, milk

MID-MORNING
Piece fruit

LUNCH
Feta and walnut salad
Grapes

MAIN MEAL
Courgette and tomato gratin
Glass of wine
Slice of bran cake

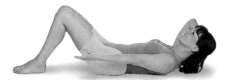

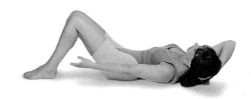

Your waist – *the forgotten bit in the middle*

1 Take up the position as shown.
Make sure the small of your
back is pressed downwards
onto the mat or carpet and that
your pelvis is tilted upwards
towards your navel. Place your
right hand under your head
(not on your neck), and look
up at the ceiling. Breathe in.

2 Breathe out and reach sideways
to your left foot. Make sure
that your right elbow is not
facing the ceiling. This is a
sideways 'swivel'. You don't
need to touch your foot –
making the effort and the
correct movement is enough to
have the right effect. Do 12
reaches on this side, rest for
20 seconds, then change hands
and repeat on the other side.

Your goal:
a total of 24 repetitions
on each side.

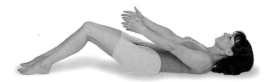

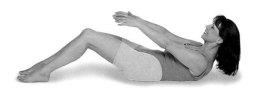

It's my stomach!

1 Take up the position as shown. Keep your knees together at all times. This is important because during the effort of abdominal exercises, the body tries to help itself by transferring the effort anywhere else it can, and that means the powerful muscles in your thighs, the quadriceps muscles. Holding your knees together renders your legs inactive. Press back downwards, breathe in and then breathe out. Cradle your head in one hand as before – don't pull on your neck – and raise your head and shoulders off the floor if you need to.

2 Stay there and breathe easily. Now, release your hand, reach forward with both hands as shown, tuck your pelvis up, press your stomach downwards and hold the position.

3 'Pulse' 6 times. Hold. Breathe in and then breathe out.

4 Bring your fingertips back to your temples and slowly release back on to the floor.

Your goal:
do 6 repetitions, rest and then do 6 again.

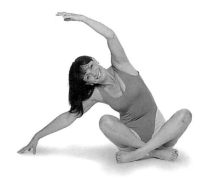

It's this bit on my hips

1 Sit cross-legged on the floor, as shown. Place your right hand on the floor and raise your left hand above your head.

2 Let the fingertips of your right hand slide slowly along the floor, a couple of centimetres at a time. Hold after every few centimetres. Breathe in and then breathe out, and let your top arm stretch over the top of your head. Keep both buttocks planted firmly on the floor and hold again. You should feel a strong stretch right down your side and into your hip. Slowly come back to the centre using your right hand to 'walk' you back to upright. Release your top arm and repeat on your other side.

Your goal:
do 3 repetitions on each side, rest and then repeat. Always do this exercise at the end of your aerobic workout.

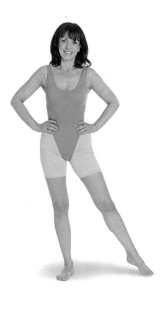

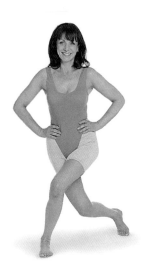

Beating those saddlebags

1 Stand upright with your feet together. Take a side step and bring one leg behind, as shown. It looks a bit like a curtsey.
2 Bring your feet back together again and repeat on the other side. Keep your hands on your hips, as in the picture, and use them for balance . As you curtsey, bring your hands to your thighs for balance. The movement is step – curtsey – step back together – curtsey on the other side, and so on.

Your goal:
do 12 repetitions on each side, rest and then repeat if possible. Stretch out afterwards, as shown in stretch 1.

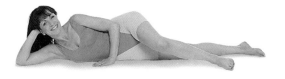

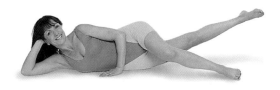

Inner thighs

1 To shape up your thighs, lie on the floor, as shown, with your top leg over your bottom leg. Now, breathe in.

2 Breathe out while you slowly raise your lower leg and hold. Try to breathe easily and don't raise your leg too high. Now stretch your toes and point them, feeling your lower leg elongating and going further. Hold for 5 seconds and then release to the floor. (The pace of this exercise should be about 6 a minute.)

Your goal:
do 10 repetitions with each leg, rest and then repeat. Stretch out, as shown in stretch 2.

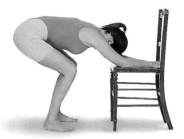

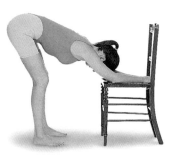

Crouching quadriceps pliés

1 With feet slightly wider than hip-distance apart, bend your knees and place your forearms on the back of a chair, as shown. Lower your hips until your knees are at right angles to the floor.

2 Raise your bottom 15–20 cm, then lower again, keeping your shoulders down by the chair. This must be done slowly, raising to a count of 4, then release to a count of 4.

Your goal:
do 12 repetitions, rest and repeat – it's hard!

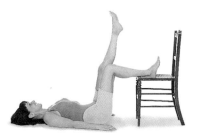

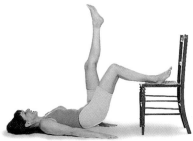

Declining hamstring bridges

1 Lie on the floor with your feet on a chair. Use both feet to start with.
2 Slowly raise your buttocks off the floor, making sure that you don't thrust your hips towards the ceiling, which would simply flex your stomach muscles. Do 16 of these.
3 In the advanced move, place one foot on your opposite thigh, or extend the leg into the air, as shown.

Your goal:
do 16 repetitions with both feet on the chair, then 12 for each single leg. Rest and repeat.

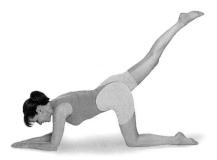

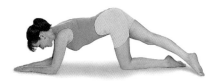

Glute sweeps

1 Take up the position, as shown, on your elbows and knees. Keep your hips square to the floor. Raise your right leg, making sure your knee is facing towards the floor and not turning outwards. Do not dip your back and keep your stomach pulled in tightly.

2 Slowly lower your right leg crossing it over the left leg and touching your toe to the floor. Raise it again slowly and make sure you squeeze your buttock tightly as you hold your leg at its highest point. Do 12 of these, rest and then change legs and repeat.

Your goal:
do 12 repetitions on each leg, rest and repeat.

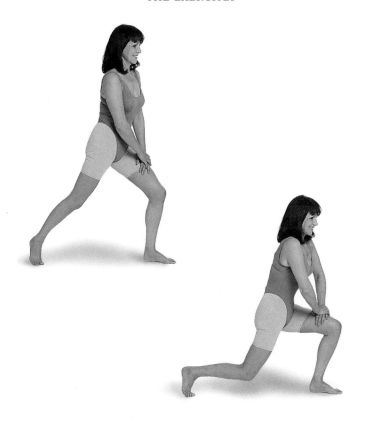

Standing dips

1 Take up the position, as
shown, with one leg behind
the other, then take a small step
to the side for balance. Lean
forwards, feeling all the effort
in your front buttock. Dip
downwards and raise yourself
again, 8 times. Change legs
and repeat.

Your goal:
do 8 repetitions on each leg,
rest and repeat. After 2 weeks
you should increase this to
3 sets on each leg.

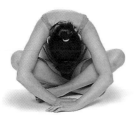

Outer thigh stretch

Sit on the floor, cross-legged, and inhale. Exhale, and slowly lean forward over your legs as shown, placing your hands on the floor and lowering your head. Hold for 10 seconds.

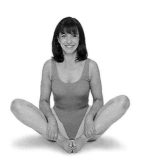

Inner thigh stretch

Sit on the floor with the soles of your feet together. Place your hands on your ankles, breathe in and lift your ribcage. Slightly lean forward, pressing your knees downwards to the floor, feeling the stretch in your inner thighs. Hold for a count of 10, release and repeat the stretch.

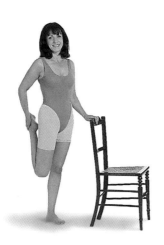

Quadriceps stretch

Stand sideways to a chair, maintaining balance with one hand. Bring one foot backwards towards your buttocks and hold. Make sure your knees are touching, your supporting leg is slightly 'soft' at the knee, and your back is not arched. Hold for a count of 20. Change legs.

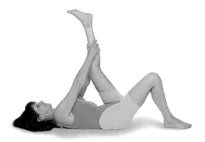

Hamstring stretch

Lie on the floor with one knee
bent, the foot flat on the floor.
Lift the other leg and hold it
behind the calf or thigh. Stretch
the leg to the ceiling as much or
as little as you can. Try not to lift
your buttocks off the floor. Hold
for a count of 20, change legs.

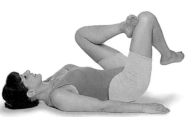

Gluteal stretch

Lie on the floor as for the hamstring stretch. Rest your arms and
hands on the floor by your sides.
Place your left foot across the
opposite knee and lift your right
foot from the floor until you feel
a stretch in your buttock. Hold
for 20 seconds, change legs.

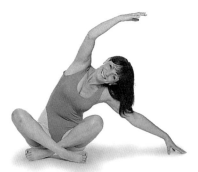

Waist stretch

Sit cross-legged on the floor.
Raise both hands above your
head. Breathe in. Keep your right
arm high, breathe out and slowly
lower your left arm until your
fingertips touch the floor. Hold,
and slowly 'walk' your fingertips
away until the stretch is strong.
Hold for a count of 10, slowly
return to the centre and relax.
Repeat on the other side.

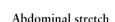

Abdominal stretch

Lie on your stomach with your
forearms flat on the floor. Breathe
in, then breathe out as you slowly
press backwards until you feel
a stretch in your abdomen. Keep
your neck in line with your back,
hold for 20 seconds, release
and repeat.

Wheat-free Menu Ideas

―――――― Day 1 ――――――

BREAKFAST
Porridge with milk
½ grapefruit

MID-MORNING
Apple

LUNCH
Chicken or cheese salad
Apple

MAIN MEAL
Stir-fried chicken and vegetables
with rice
Piece of fruit

―――――― Day 2 ――――――

BREAKFAST
Small bowl of porridge with 150
ml skimmed milk., topped with
½ chopped apple

MID-MORNING
1 apple, small bunch grapes

LUNCH
Cold chicken served on 2 tbsp
potato salad with a green salad
and cold peas and 1 tbsp
vinaigrette dressing
1 banana

MAIN MEAL
Poached salmon with salad
Portion roasted pineapple with
crème fraîche

―――――― Day 3 ――――――

BREAKFAST
2 scrambled eggs, 3 rashers of
bacon
Glass of fresh orange juice

MID-MORNING
Apple

LUNCH
Large mixed winter salad

MAIN MEAL
Spicy yoghurt-baked chicken
with rice
Salad or vegetables

―――――― Day 4 ――――――

BREAKFAST
Rice Krispies and milk with
banana
(permitted breakfast cereal for
wheat-free menus)

MID-MORNING
Grapes

LUNCH
Cottage cheese and 3-fruit salad

MAIN MEAL
Smoked salmon on potato cakes
Salad or broccoli

———— Day 5 ————

BREAKFAST
Porridge with milk

MID-MORNING
1 piece fruit

LUNCH
Waldorf salad

DINNER
Roast chicken or beef with
    mashed parsnips, carrots and
    3 boiled potatoes
Fresh fruit salad with crème
    fraîche

———— Day 6 ————

BREAKFAST
2 scrambled eggs on 1 slice of rye
    toast
Bowl grapefruit segments

LUNCH
Spinach and avocado salad
Apple

MAIN MEAL
Jacket potato with tuna and
    salad
2 scoops ice cream
1 glass wine

———— Day 7 ————

BREAKFAST
3-fruit salad including banana,
    with yoghurt

MID-MORNING
Nothing

LUNCH
Salade Niçoise

MAIN MEAL
2-egg omelette with salad and
    a jacket potato

Menus for Snackers

Sometimes your schedule – or your cooking facilities – just
won't allow for fancy menus. But snackers beware! You are the
most likely to be eating way over your CarboRange because

snack food tends to be high-carbohydrate. These menu plans are all under 150 carbograms a day, so should help you to stay on track.

─────── Day 1 ───────

BREAKFAST
Two Shredded Wheat with milk

MID-MORNING
Satsuma

LUNCH
Slice of bran cake
Apple

LIGHT EVENING SNACK
2 tbsp baked beans on 1 slice of
   toast
Grapes

SUPPER
Handful of nuts and raisins
Apple

─────── Day 2 ───────

BREAKFAST
2 slices of toast and marmalade

MID-MORNING
Apple and banana

LUNCH
Waldorf Salad

LIGHT EVENING MEAL
Poached salmon salad (bought)
Glass of wine

SUPPER
2 apples
Chewy cereal bar

─────── Day 3 ───────

BREAKFAST
Glass of fresh orange juice
Banana

MID-MORNING
Apple

LUNCH
Large mixed winter salad

LIGHT EVENING MEAL
Slice of pizza with salad
Piece of fruit

─────── Day 4 ───────

BREAKFAST
Bowl of muesli with milk and
   sliced apple

MID-MORNING
Pot yoghurt

LUNCH
Tub of cottage cheese with
   banana and grapes

LIGHT EVENING MEAL
Chicken stir-fry

SUPPER
Round of salad sandwiches

——————— Day 5 ———————

BREAKFAST
Cereal with milk

MID-MORNING
1 piece of fruit

LUNCH
Pitta bread with hummus

LIGHT EVENING MEAL
Pasta with vegetable sauce

SUPPER
Banana and a small bag of nuts
and raisins

——————— Day 6 ———————

BREAKFAST
Fresh fruit salad

MID-MORNING
Banana and 3 Brazil nuts

LUNCH
Submarine roll filled with chicken
tikka and salad
Apple

LIGHT EVENING MEAL
Stir-fry chicken or fish with
mixed vegetables
1 glass of wine

——————— Day 7 ———————

BREAKFAST
Banana milkshake

MID-MORNING
Pear

LUNCH
Tuna fish sandwich with salad
Apple

LIGHT EVENING MEAL
Slice of quiche with salad
Strawberries and 1 scoop of ice
cream

Very-Low-Carbohydrate Diet

This is not recommended for people with an active lifestyle. But
if you have a thyroid condition, for example, or are inactive or
recovering after a period of illness, you will need fewer carbo-

hydrates. These menus all supply good nutrition but very low carbohydrates. I have not given carbogram values, but the menus are all below 100. Do not follow them for more than 4 weeks without a week off.

--------- Day 1 ---------

BREAKFAST
Cereal and milk with ½ apple, sliced

LUNCH
Ham or cheese salad
Banana
Apple

MAIN MEAL
Roast chicken or beef, or a plain grilled chop, with 3 green vegetables, no potatoes
Baked pear with 1 tbsp yoghurt or crème fraîche

--------- Day 2 ---------

BREAKFAST
Scrambled eggs with 1 slice of toast
Bowl grapefruit segments

LUNCH
Cottage cheese and fruit salad

MAIN MEAL
Poached cod or salmon with peas, asparagus and broccoli and a light parsley sauce
Roast pineapple and crème fraîche or yoghurt

--------- Day 3 ---------

BREAKFAST
Muesli with milk

LUNCH
Cheese salad
Apple

MAIN MEAL
3 slices cold meat or ½ tin tuna fish with salad
Banana and 1 tbsp low-fat custard
Glass of wine

--------- Day 4 ---------

BREAKFAST
2 poached eggs and 2 rashers bacon
Small glass of fresh orange juice

LUNCH
Winter salad, banana

MAIN MEAL
Portion of chilli con carne or curry with grated carrot instead of rice
Mixed fruit salad with 1 tbsp yoghurt

Day 5

BREAKFAST

Kippers or 2 Weetabix and milk

LUNCH

½ avocado with smoked salmon
  or stick of cheese with an apple

MAIN MEAL

Poached cod in caper sauce with
  broccoli, carrots and French
  beans, no rice
Hot spiced oranges
Glass of wine

Day 6

BREAKFAST

Special K with milk
Apple

LUNCH

Cottage cheese and fruit platter
  or cottage cheese with 4
  crispbreads

MAIN MEAL

Courgette and tomato gratin
Grilled chicken
Slice roast pineapple or a
  caramelized pear

Day 7

BREAKFAST

Omelette and 1 slice of toast and
  marmalade

LUNCH

Feta and walnut salad (or use any
  cheese)

MAIN MEAL

3 slices of roast meat or a small
  steak with salad or 3
  vegetables
Small pot chocolate mousse
2 glasses of wine

High-CarboRange Meals

For special occasion days you need a high-CarboRange meal. This means saving up your carbograms for that one meal – but all the same you must have breakfast and you must have four pieces of fruit during the day. High-CarboRange meals are not a good idea too often for two reasons: first, you are trying to train your appetite and habits so you eat regularly spaced meals every day; second, if this meal is in the evening, it is a lot of calories to eat just a couple of hours before bedtime – anything up to 1,000 or 1,200.

However, we all go out for meals like these and it is unrealistic to expect you not to join in with everyone else. I have given some meal examples here which give you a good idea of how the carbograms stack up.

If someone is cooking for you it is virtually impossible to count carbograms accurately. Try to get acquainted with carbograms so you know the best way to avoid high-carbogram foods like puddings, bread and cakes and it will still be easy to stay within your diet budget.

Menu ideas: all around 100 carbograms

MEAL ONE
Salmon fillet with sauté potatoes, 3 vegetables and salad
2 scoops of ice cream
2 glasses of dry white wine
Coffee with two after-dinner mints

MEAL TWO
Whole pan pizza and a side salad
2 scoops of ice cream
1 glass of red wine

87

MEAL THREE
Steak and kidney pie, 200g portion with boiled potatoes and 2
   vegetables
Slice of cheesecake
2 glasses of wine

MEAL FOUR
Roast chicken, 2 roast potatoes, 3 vegetables, stuffing, gravy,
   bread sauce and cranberry sauce
Apple pie with pastry

MEAL FIVE
Bread roll and butter
Slice of melon
Steak with salad and sauté potatoes
Chocolate cream dessert
2 glasses of dry white wine
Coffee

MEAL SIX
Any meat or vegetable curry and a poppadom
Portion of ice cream
Pint of lager

MEAL SEVEN
2 slices of olive bread with olive oil
Avocado with prawns or crabmeat and salad
Roast lamb or poached or roasted fish with roasted vegetables
Crème brulée
2 glasses of wine
Coffee with petit fours

Keeping Your Meals Out Low-carbogram
Meals out need not bust your carbogram budget. Here's how to
do it:

- Avoid the bread – even nibbling at a piece uses 10–20cg.
- Hold the potatoes – you can have extra vegetables and even more meat or fish.
- Choose fresh fruit puddings for just 30cg.
- Have dry alcoholic drink rather than sweet, to save 3cg a time.
- Watch the accompaniments – bread sauce is high in starch, cranberry sauce is high in sugar.
- Be careful of added carbohydrates like thickened soups or sweetened puddings. These have a massive carbogram penalty.

Shaping Back Into Those Jeans

People groan whenever they hear the word 'exercise'. It conjures up images of hard-faced aerobics queens, sweaty games of squash, or tying themselves up in knots at yoga classes. But it doesn't have to be like that.

The distribution of your weight is as important to your looks as what you weigh. To a certain extent it's down to genetics, but a lot of your shape is also determined by the way you live. Sitting down spreads your bottom and thighs, while manual work can build up your shoulders. Hairdressers develop sway backs and protruding stomachs. All these problems can be helped by regular toning exercise which you should do in your own home as regularly as you would wash your hair.

There are five ways in which you can change your shape:

First Gear – Getting Going

Everyday exercise

You get exercise every time you make a movement. Think back to where we discussed your basal metabolic rate (BMR). If you remember, your BMR is based on the calories that your body would use if you were doing nothing. Think of it as a car engine idling, with the speedometer needle set at zero. You put the car into first gear and then begin to move slowly. The needle moves up to five miles an hour and then ten. You change gear, gather speed until you are in top gear at seventy miles an hour and the engine is burning a lot of fuel. Well, your body is like that. From the moment you wake up, your needle is slowly going up. You get out of bed and go downstairs, you make tea and feed the cat. By doing this, you have gathered speed. You have gone from burning one calorie a minute to one and a half. Throughout the day you will be changing gear and either burning more fuel, such as in a brisk run for the train, or slowing down, as you might do by sitting at your office desk. Life may seem hectic in your head, but sitting down at a desk all day burns very few calories. By lunchtime each day, most sedentary workers have consumed far more calories than they have burned off.

Life used to be active because people didn't have the range of labour-saving devices and machines available today. Now we press a switch and flick a button, and our work's done. Compare this with the old days of preparing supper, which would involve washing and peeling vegetables, grating and chopping, and going in and out of the back door to dispose of leftovers. My mother used to be in the kitchen for the whole of Sunday making lunch and tea, but nowadays we put a ready-made meat and two veg meal into the microwave and it's done in minutes. Salads come in hygienic, no-waste packs, and vegetables are completely prepared for us right down to the cross in the bottom of a sprout. The trouble is: three hours of work was a lot of calories. It's no wonder people get fat when they purchase a dishwasher and give up over two hours of washing-up each week.

I'm not suggesting that we go back to those days – I use a dishwasher too – but if you've outgrown those jeans you need to do something. Just to get you into the swing of things, I have compiled this fun-chart which counts the calories of everyday tasks:

Calories used in a year

Activity	Calories Used	The Old Way	Calories Used
Changing TV channels with remote control three times in an evening	1,095	Getting up to change channels	2,190
Having someone else make you coffee twice a day, five days a week	1,920	Walking 100 yards to make your own coffee	4,800
Washing your car in a car wash (once a week)	156	Washing your car by hand (thirty minutes)	4,160
Taking your shopping 100 yards to your car in a trolley	600	Carrying heavy shopping to your car twice a week	1,200
Sitting in front of the TV for ten minutes, seven nights a week	3,650	Going for a ten-minute walk seven times a week	18,250
Driving or riding in the bus the whole distance, five days a week, forty-eight weeks a year	240	Parking or alighting five minutes away from your stop and walking the rest of the way (there and back)	12,000
Total:	7,661		42,600

The chart may be for fun, but it is also accurate. These simple tasks add up to a staggering 34,939 *extra* calories used in a year, which is a whole four kilos' worth of fat!

Your goal

You should aim to burn off an extra 150 calories a day through normal activities such as the following:

- fifteen minutes' hand washing
- getting up an hour earlier
- a ten-minute brisk walk to post a letter and back
- eight minutes spent raking leaves or brisk sweeping

Second Gear – Burning Those Calories

Monica's motto

'If it moves, nothing can settle.' Fat loves little corners where it won't be disturbed, so *keep everything moving*! Burning away those calories and fat is what you want to achieve, and you can only do this effectively with aerobic exercise.

Aerobic means 'with air' and it encompasses all the activities that make you slightly breathless and with a faster heartbeat. If you were aiming to be an elite sportsperson I would be talking about percentages of your body's maximum heart rate and volumes of air, but you don't need to worry too much about those sorts of details simply to get back into your jeans! You just want to slice those inches off your thighs and bottom, and one of the most effective ways to deal with fat is through aerobic exercise. The chart that follows lists all the advantages of aerobic exercise, as well as what it can't achieve.

What aerobic exercise *does*	What it *doesn't do*
• increases heart rate	• change the shapes of your muscles
• improves circulation	• make your muscles leaner
• burns calories	• make you more flexible
• gives you more stamina	
• tones muscles, especially in the lower body	

The best activities for calorie-burning are those which are moderate and long-lasting. Short, hard exercise such as a sprint or racing swimming cannot be endured for hours on end, so although the calories burned are greater per minute than for more moderate exercise, the simple fact that you can go on for longer in exercise such as step aerobics, slow swimming or a day's rambling means that more calories are burned and your system is more efficient.

Turning back to the analogy of a car going through its gears, reaching top gear and settling down into a long motorway run is fuel-efficient and relaxing for the driver. The car works at its best at less than top speed, and so do you. Short, sharp bursts of fast driving cannot be prolonged: they use a lot of fuel and cause wear and tear.

If you're going to get the best from your body you're not going to do it by short, hard games of squash after a day of sitting down. They might exhaust you, but they don't use your fuel efficiently. You need to get into your stride by cycling to work, walking the dog for an afternoon at the weekend or getting on that treadmill and walking briskly for forty-five minutes. Your metabolism stays high for a long time afterwards and this matters in weight control and fat burning. In short, sharp bursts you recover quickly, but at the end of longer bouts of moderate exercise your energy supplies are completely out.

Eating at this stage is the best way of using your food because it replenishes what you've lost. Unless you eat a really gigantic meal it won't be stored as fat, simply because there won't be anything left as excess.

If you get your exercise in the gym, vary your work-outs between the stairclimber, cycle and treadmill. As you improve and get fitter, don't just make the work-outs longer: make them more intense. Many people can only spare forty-five minutes in the gym at any one time and they cheerfully stick with the same routine, year after year, on auto-pilot. They stagger into the gym half asleep, go through their work-out programme, shower and go to work. There is no thought of testing the boundaries, no consideration of variation or intensity. The fact is, if you only have forty-five minutes then that's no problem. As you get fitter and more used to your routine, increase the intensity and not the time spent in the gym. Get the treadmill to climb hills and do the same with the bike, row faster, increase the resistance on the stairclimber. You shouldn't go flat out but you should adjust your work-out. After all, you're fitter now than you used to be!

Here are some basic calorie values:

Basic calories used in exercise

Activity	Calories used per half hour
Walking slowly	120
Walking briskly	180
Walking uphill	240
Playing tennis	210
Jogging	240
Squash	420
Ice skating	150
Aerobics – high impact	195
Aerobics – low impact	165

Activity	Calories used per half hour
Gentle cycling	120
Fast cycling	195
Racing cycling	330
Disco dancing	195
Ballroom dancing	105
Golf	165
Horse riding, trotting	210
Netball	210
Slow swimming	255
Fast swimming	300
Medium-paced running	375

Your goal

The aim is to burn off an *extra* 150 calories a day with an aerobic activity or sport. Here is an example:

Monday	Low-impact aerobics class
Tuesday	Walk to work or have an evening walk
Wednesday	Day off
Thursday	Twenty-minute swim at lunchtime
Friday	Morning or evening walk
Saturday	Game of squash, tennis, football, etc.
Sunday	Cycle ride

Arrange your activities in any way that suits you, but try to get that half hour or so of aerobic exercise on six days of the week. Amazingly, that little bit extra adds up to a staggering 144 *hours*, or six *whole days* of exercise a year, and an even more amazing 43,200 calories, which is 5.5 kilos (12lb) of your weight gone for good!

What, you don't believe me? Sounds like just a theory? Don't forget that not following this sort of pattern is how your weight crept on in the first place. Take a desk job or give up a manual job for home life and it's a slow decline in activity. Half an hour a day, three hours a week of not being active means that you aren't using up 1,000 calories a week. It all adds up, and suddenly those jeans won't fasten. It's as simple as that.

Third Gear – Toning For A Better Shape

You've burned off fat, but if you're not careful you could end up looking like a rag doll without its stuffing. Fat and muscle are completely different things which simply share a home and, as I said earlier, don't assume your weight is all unwelcome fat. Unless you actually have a fat monitoring machine (and they can be bought in branches of the larger chemists' stores) you won't know how much of your weight is healthy muscle and how much is fat. To give you an idea of how fooled we can be about our fitness, the maximum recommended healthy fat reading for women is 29 per cent. Now, I have a friend, a twig of 51 kilos (8 stone) who commends herself on never taking any exercise. But according to my fat monitor she registered a worrying 38 per cent fat! Yes, she was slim, but at the same time unhealthily fat. We have now embarked on a programme to help her lose the fat and replace the weight, while filling out her skin with healthy and atttractive-looking muscle.

Toning exercise firms up your muscles, makes them longer and stronger, and gives them definition. It is carried out using your body's own weight – for example, in leg lifts where you are raising your leg against its own weight, which could be as much as 6.5 kilos (14lb). Toning increases muscle fibres slightly and you will achieve a firmer thigh, a tighter bottom, a flatter stomach and a slimmer waist. Here are the areas you need to work to get back into those jeans:

1 waist
2 stomach
3 'love handles' – the top of the hip bones
4 inner thighs
5 outer thighs
6 front of thighs
7 backs of thighs
8 bottom

I shall be dividing your exercises into two groups, which you work on alternate days for balance (see pages 104–6), and to give muscle groups time to recover and improve.

Fourth Gear – Sculpting

'Sculpting' is quite a new term. In reality it is simply weight training, but therein lies a problematic image of muscle-bound, hard-faced women with mahogany tans and oiled bodies – fairly off-putting to a lot of us!

But don't be put off. Sculpting is something I do, and I am quite small and not remotely hefty. It means the use of heavier weights for shorter periods of time to increase the size of a particular muscle or to improve its shape, and I have followed a programme for two years now to help improve the appearance of my shoulders and arms. Using weights on your legs won't necessarily make them bigger, if you know just how far to go. What they will do, without gaining any extra size, is make your legs amazingly tight and hard.

If you really get into a sculpting programme you can say goodbye to any wobble or splay effect. 'Splay' is what happens when you force yourself into too-tight jeans and your spare buttocks splay out to make 'saddlebags'. In your jeans, your bottom will look fantastic!

Someone who went through this plan to test it for me became the envy of her whole office. 'I couldn't believe it,' said a friend, 'there wasn't a bulge anywhere. Her bum was smooth under her jeans with no hint of a droop!' This improvement came about purely through sculpting exercise.

How it works
Muscle gets bigger by growing more fibres. It does this because it is being forced to work under increasing weights and in resting periods your muscles produce these extra fibres. You can prevent your body from forming huge muscles by limiting the weights you use and stretching your muscles after your work-out.

Don't forget, the more muscle you have the higher your resting metabolic rate – and the more efficiently you will be burning off calories.

The warm-up
Always warm up for a few minutes first by walking on the spot or stepping from side to side, swinging your arms, or you could cycle on a stationary bike for five minutes. Stretch out afterwards.

Your waist – the forgotten bit in the middle
There is one simple exercise for your waist which you do lying on the floor, which you will find in the photo section.

This exercise is effective because it is a stretching movement which tones the oblique muscles. (They run along the side of your torso and shape your waist.)

It's my stomach!
If you haven't already got my book *5 Days to a Flatter Stomach*, then rush out and buy it now because it has some lovely exercises for you to get your teeth into on this month's plan. It

also has specific advice on the other causes of a problem stomach, some of which you may not already have thought of. However, working the stomach can be done with one simple exercise – as long as you promise yourself to do it every day, do all the repetitions and stick with the rules of correct form. You'll find it in the photo section.

This exercise is so slow that as a guide, you should do no more than four repetitions in a minute.

It's this bit on my hips

How many times have I heard that? People come up to me holding bits of flesh with a look of utter despair on their faces, yet that little fleshy 'pad' on the top of your pelvic bones seems to defy all attempts to shift it. And the reason? This area simply doesn't get to move very much in daily life and, as I keep on saying, fat loves little corners where it knows it won't be disturbed.

There is one exercise which I swear by to whittle down that pad and it is, in fact, a stretch. Stick with it. At first you may feel a little stiff the next day and you may also feel that it isn't doing anything – but it is. The stiffness is caused by the muscles in your back and your hips being stretched really thoroughly, probably for the first time. It takes time because these things do. You wouldn't expect your hair to grow back in one week if you'd had it cut too short, and neither will your body change shape miraculously. But by the end of this month, you'll notice a huge difference. Have a look at the instructions in the picture section.

This exercise is hard to do and you mustn't feel discouraged if you can't go very far. It will come.

Beating those saddlebags

I can think of more than a dozen exercises for your outer thighs, but my clients have always told me that nothing worked better than my own invention, an exercise I call the 'curtsey'. It's in the picture section.

It's not easy, but if you are a complete beginner you can do the simpler version, which is just as effective, and then work up to the full effort. The reason why this movement works so well is because you have to use each leg to raise your whole body weight. I can promise you that when it comes to trimming outer thighs to get back into your jeans, this exercise is the business!

It's best to have some music for this, something which has about 100 beats to the minute. Try to find a suitable piece because it's going to be very useful in the weeks ahead.

Inner thighs

Most of us are unhappy about the shape of our inner thighs. Like hips, they can get out of condition because they are not used very much. The inner thigh muscles are called 'adductors' and they only work when you draw your legs together – not something we do very often! Gripping movements with your thighs, such as in horse riding, are excellent for toning the adductors, but if you are not into riding then you need to make a special effort to tone them.

To get rid of fat on the inner thighs, I recommend the following types of exercise:

- fast swimming
- aerobics
- ballroom dancing
- ballet
- tennis
- football

If you want to shape up flabby, but slim, inner thighs, try the following:

- floor exercises
- horse riding
- stretching

Fronts of thighs
If you want to lose weight from large thighs, try the following:

- fast cycling
- swimming
- dancing
- brisk walking

To shape up untoned slim legs, try the following:

- floor exercises adding light (450g–1.5kg) ankle weights
- stretching
- mountain or resistance cycling
- step aerobics
- leg extensions (in the gym)
- lunges and squats (see below for one version)

Crouching quadricep pliés
This is not the most elegant of exercises – but so what? You're in the privacy of your own home and can look as silly as you like. After all, you won't look so silly when the zip on those jeans glides up effortlessly, and all your friends are whispering about your fantastic thighs! The instructions are on **page vi** of the photo section.

Backs of thighs
The hamstrings run along the backs of your thighs. Toning them gives an impressive sweep to the backs of your legs and helps to prevent cellulite from developing. The exercise in the photo section is easy for everyone, although it does take prac-

tice. Do as many as you can, going on to the advanced form of the exercise as you get stronger.

The bottom line – 'glute sweeps'

Your buttock muscles are called 'gluteals' or 'glutes' for short. They are big muscles and they can get out of shape and become slack very quickly. If you stand or sit a lot of the time, you may need firming exercises if you want to have a firm, high bottom.

As with thighs, fast cycling, swimming, skating or hill walking are good fat burners, but toning work to really strengthen and lift the buttocks should be done with resistance. Try any of the following, or the Glute Sweeps in the photo section.

- hill or mountain cycling
- step aerobics
- lunges
- squats
- skiing squats
- Standing Dips

'Glute bridges'

This exercise can be done by old and young alike, while you're on the telephone or watching TV. If you like, place a 1.5–4.5 kilo weight on your hips. It tones and tightens the buttock muscles. Although it's not photographed, it's very straightforward. Lie on the floor, knees bent, feet flat on the floor. Being careful not to arch your back or thrust your pelvis into the air, lift your buttocks just clear of the floor. Squeeze and release them at a rate of once a second. Try to do 20 with knees touching, 20 with knees apart, and 20 with heels only on the floor, toes raised!

Back To Neutral Gear – Stretching Out

Now it's time to cool your engine down and to come back to where you started. You've burned off a lot of calories and they will continue to be burned for one to two hours if you've done vigorous exercise which has lasted over an hour. Stretching ensures a nice long, lean line to your body and this is essential if you are to achieve your goal of getting back into those jeans. Never underestimate the value of stretching. It is as important to losing weight as diet or aerobics (see photo section).

1 Outer Thigh Stretch
2 Inner Thigh Stretch
3 Quadriceps Stretch
4 Hamstring Stretch
5 Gluteal Stretch
6 Waist Stretch
7 Abdominal Stretch

Devising a fitness programme for your whole body

When you start your exercise programme, it's easy to be positive and motivated. By the end of a couple of weeks, though, this enthusiasm has often waned. You haven't shrunk two sizes, you haven't lost a stone, you're exhausted and you wonder if it's worth it.

There are two reasons for feeling like this. Going at an exercise programme like a bull at a gate is one thing, and following the same routine day after day is another. However tempted you might be to exercise for two hours a day – don't. Working out a long-term programme means that you won't just stay interested for longer, but you'll reprogramme your body and maintain your fitness level even when resting. Here is an ideal programme to follow:

First Week

Monday
Early morning walk
Aerobics class in the evening or sports session
Floor exercises at home or in the gym:

> Inner Thighs
> Outer Thighs ('Curtseys' of photo section)
> Crouching Pliés (for fronts of thighs of photo section)
> Stomach
> Waist Reaches

Tuesday
Early morning walk *or* thirty minutes on the treadmill at 4 m.p.h.
Swimming at lunchtime or in the evening
Floorwork:

> Glute Sweeps
> Glute Bridges (see **page 103**)
> Standing Dips
> Hip Stretch
> Stomach

   In the second week, start to use weights to make the exercises
a little harder!

Wednesday
This is your day off. Have a walk or easy cycle ride, if possible.

Thursday
Bike ride for forty-five minutes *or* forty-five minutes' brisk or
hill walking *or* forty-five minutes on a treadmill at 4.2 m.p.h.
   Floorwork, as Monday.

Friday
Thirty minutes early morning walk
Thirty minutes exercise bike (if available) *or* thirty minutes on the stairclimber.

At lunchtime, either walk, swim or go to an exercise class.

Floorwork, as Tuesday.

Saturday
This is your full day off.

Sunday
Full programme: forty-five minutes on an exercise bike *or* a cycle ride. Thirty minutes walking (4.5 m.p.h.) *or* use the stairclimber.

These should all be carried out at moderate pace, with no running or jogging.

Floorwork: a full programme of *all* the exercises, with full sets of repetitions.

Second Week
1 Repeat the programme as for last week allowing a full day off after each two days of exercise.
2 Start to add 450g weights to your ankles for inner thigh exercises, hold weights on hips for Glute Bridges (see page 103).
3 Don't forget to warm up and do a full stretch session after every work-out.

What Next?

Managing Your Shape For The Future

Earlier, I talked about the difference between a results diet and a lifestyle diet. Now that you have lost the excess weight, it is time to decide which one you want. I have a diet that works for me. You need to devise a personal diet, based, I hope, on the carbogram system, which takes into account not just the foods you like, but the fact that you sometimes find eating a bit of a temptation!

Your style of eating and the things you eat are your diet and, as far as I know, every smart woman has her own personal diet style.

Having to watch what you eat is no worse than having to watch your hair or having to be careful about your nails. Looking good always has and always will be an effort. People who make no effort show it. Although I have promised you that no foods are banned, I know you're only human. If you know that once you open that packet of custard creams all hell breaks loose, don't buy them. Life won't stop if you never see the inside of a chip shop again or only savour a prawn vindaloo on your birthday. In any case, it's not that bad. Just keep those foods for special occasions, and you'll appreciate them all the more. You have the willpower, and you have it because you've come this far and the pleasure you'll get from all the compliments about your new figure will far outweigh the fleeting excitement of a bit of cake.

Your new regime can be more relaxed because you are

familiar with carbohydrates and don't need to walk around with the book in your pocket. Add carbograms if you want to, but don't bargain with your body. Adding a sandwich or a serving of potatoes is a normal and natural way of enhancing an already tasty meal: adding extra alcohol, scoops of ice cream and a scattering of low-carbohydrate biscuits throughout the day simply takes you back to where you were before – treating food as a filler and eating chaotically. *Don't do it!!*

Calculating Your New Carbohydrate Allowance

You can now choose more carbograms. Your personal needs depend on your weight and the amount of activity you engage in. But on this occasion you need to calculate according to the weight you *want to be*. Start with your weight in kilos and follow the table below according to your general level of activity.

Activity Level	Grams of Carbohydrate Per kg of Weight
Light (less than an hour a day)	3–4
Moderate (1–2 hours a day)	4–5
Heavy (2–4 hours a day)	5–6

Note:

Light	Standing or sitting all day, driving, craftwork, light housework, cooking.
Moderate	Walking to and from school or work, shopping, gardening, keep-fit class.
Heavy	Competitive sports, walking for a living (e.g. traffic warden, beat police officer, postman), mountain biking, daily horse riding.

Therefore if you are 70 kilos but want to be 64 kilos (10.5 stone), and you are doing an office job, you would need 63 x 3 grams of carbohydrate a day, which comes to 192 grams.

How Do I Know How Much Carbohydrate Is In My Food?

Just read the food labels! I have prepared this handy guide to the most common foods that we eat with typical portion sizes. Don't worry, you won't spend the rest of your life weighing and counting. After a while you'll have a good idea of portion sizes even if there isn't a pair of scales in sight.

These food portions all contain 25cg:

1–2 slices bread	1–2 Weetabix
150g potatoes	40g muesli
75g cooked rice	568ml milk
2 bananas	2–3 apples
150g baked beans	Half slice fruit cake
2–3 oranges	284ml orange juice
2–3 small cartons plain yoghurt	2 bowls (60g) porridge
50g raisins	90g cooked pasta
115g sweetcorn	2 packets crisps
25g chocolate	150g cooked noodles
150g butter beans	140g lentils
4 slices Ryvita	3 tsp honey

So, with an allowance of 192cg, you could make eight choices from this list and add your protein foods.

Sample menus

Breakfast: Muesli, milk, apple

Lunch: Tuna fish sandwich, banana, packet crisps

Snack: Apple and banana

Main meal: Jacket potato, ham, mixed bean salad, small slice fruit cake, coffee.

Total = 198g of carbohydrate, and 1,498 calories.

Breakfast: Bacon, egg, two slices of bread and butter

Lunch: Coronation Chicken, rice salad, 25g chocolate

Snack: Salad sandwich

Main meal: Lentil and Carrot Soup, Vegetable Lasagne, Fruit Salad.

Total = 197g carbohydrate and 1,682 calories.

And Finally . . .

I hope you've got back into those old jeans, or that suit or your wedding dress. And I hope you're more confident because of it and will carry on your good work for the future. Look after your new figure. Don't get obsessed about it because it will take care of itself if you remember the golden rules for lasting success:

1 Never ignore hunger. It is your body's way of telling you that it needs food for a reason.
2 Never deal with hunger by putting it off with a fizzy drink. Have some starch, such as a slice of bread, instead.
3 Never go beyond being full. Put your plate aside and leave it.

A better solution is to take a smaller portion in the first place, and add small second helpings if you need them or if it is appropriate to keep another diner company as a courtesy.

4 Never go to bed hungry.

5 Never confuse wanting to eat with being hungry. If you have eaten recently then your stomach isn't empty and you are craving food for another reason. Maybe you're bored or lonely? Next time it happens, don't have fruit, try having bread instead.

6 Exercise every day, even if it's just a walk. Think of ways to do extra exercise, such as gardening, going to post a letter or a bit of cleaning – even ten minutes a day adds up.

7 Keep supple with bending and stretching exercises (see the photo section).

8 Believe in yourself. No one was born beautiful. If someone looks beautiful it's because he/she looks after themselves. No one has a great body by accident and if you make the same effort you can look great too. It isn't easy but it *is* simple. There's no great mystery to eating less and taking a bit more exercise.

Go for it – and the very best of luck!

'It Was Brilliant!'

As always, I asked a team of volunteers to test out *The New Get Back Into Your Jeans Diet* for me. I was fortunate enough to be able to appeal for testers to try it out through my *Sunday Mirror* column and had offers from all over the country. I finally asked 100 people to tell me honestly what they thought. My aim was not simply to find out if they had lost weight, but also if the diet was practical. After all, I have said that there's a diet out there to suit everybody and in this book I have given you as many options as possible. But at the end of the day, could the volunteers take the food to work, was the whole family able to share meals, and did they find it a chore to keep records?

For the purpose of a more balanced test, twelve of the volunteers were put on a very different type of diet that was also practical and manageable. But *The New Get Back Into Your Jeans Diet* proved far and away the most successful and more significant – and the most popular one. Hear what the volunteers had to say:

Eileen, forty-three, is a community midwife in Gloucester

'I was sceptical at first. Being a midwife I am always on the move, and I wasn't sure about being able to keep a diary and look up carbograms. But I felt unfit and needed to lose about 2 stone [12 kilos], so I thought I'd give it a go. The most extraordinary thing for me was discovering how much I'd been eating! I didn't like weighing things at first but I can see now that it's absolutely essential. Thirty grams of breakfast cereal is less than you think, and I must have been having more than 100 grams before, thinking it was a normal portion. I didn't like having to restrict my fruit because I eat tons of it usually, but it made me really savour it. In the old days I'd munch an apple while driving and not even remember eating it.

'This diet made me aware of what I was eating and now I don't have to write down anything at all. In one month I went down from a size 16 to a 14, and now I've lost another 6 pounds [2.75 kilos] in the second month. My aim was to get back into a favourite holiday dress, and I can! I'm absolutely thrilled.'

Jenni, twenty-three, is a research scientist in Cambridge

'It was brilliant. I'd gained weight very quickly since getting this job a year ago, I think because of all the standing around I do now, whereas before I was quite active. I hadn't appreciated how the lack of exercise mounted up with time, especially as I don't really eat a lot. I suppose I thought I was slim for life.

'I really took the exercise message on board, and tried to increase it by starting to walk to work. I decided to stop having my newspaper delivered and now walk to the shop for it each morning. The diet was terrific because it made me decide what to eat for a week in advance, so I went to the shops with a proper list and didn't deviate from it, or eat unnecessarily "on the hoof". I knew I should be doing that anyway, but you don't always think about it, do you? I used to go home and then wonder what to eat and the cupboard would be bare so I'd pop out for a takeaway. Now I have a lot of home-made food ready-prepared in the fridge. I've lost a stone [6 kilos] in one month, and I'll never go back to the way I was before. I feel so good.'

Elsa, sixty-two, is a retired supervisor from County Down
'I have very bad arthritis so I can't exercise. I'm housebound so meals mean a lot to me. A lot of diets suggest ready-made meals, but I can't buy them where I live and I really don't want fast food as I still enjoy cooking.

'The diet worked because, as a low-energy person, I still had a nice plateful of food but not the carbohydrates. I love vegetables and salads, and often had a salad as a snack, with cheese or an egg, and this only used a few of my carbograms. I used to feel guilty about having a sandwich late in the evening, but I saved my carbograms for it and still lost weight. I've been able to get back into my favourite skirt and although I only lost 3 kilos my clothes are really loose, and that's what counts.'

Helene is thirty-two and a housewife in Cardiff
'I get pretty frazzled having five children under the age of ten. To be honest, I think trying to cope with having a coherent plan

for looking after myself is why I was so fat. I ate all the time. I found it really hard to stick with the *Get Back Into Your Jeans Diet* at first, simply because I am used to putting bits of food into my mouth all the time. I nearly gave up. After a week, though, I understood what Monica meant about retraining yourself. My first reactions were really just withdrawal symptoms. As soon as I realized all that eating was just a habit, and that my weight was going down, I felt much more positive. I lost 12 pounds [5.5 kilos] in the month and increased my exercise a lot. I've got back into my jeans which I didn't think I ever would again. They didn't fit on my thighs before, but now they're loose. I can't tell you how good it feels to be a mum of five getting back into the jeans I wore before I had the children!'

Janis, forty, is a personal finance adviser from York

'What I am most pleased about is the way my body has toned up. I didn't think a few exercises at home would make any difference, but even my husband has commented on my firmer bottom and slimmer stomach. I'm over the moon! I didn't necessarily want to lose much weight, but I knew I was eating rubbish and felt tired all the time, and had a feeling a sensible diet like this would be a real bonus. I feel great and ready for anything – so full of life. I'd recommend this diet and exercise plan to anyone.'

Anita, twenty-four, is a marketing manager from Jersey

'This was the best diet I've ever been on. It was brilliant! Although I had to think about it, I also felt that the hassle had been taken out of it by the carbohydrates being counted and the portions laid out. I admit that I have a lot of weight to lose as I'm over 17 stone [102 kilos] and want to be a size 12, but this plan gave me so much encouragement. I always thought it would be impossible for me to aim so high, but now I know

I can. I used to wonder why I kept a favourite suit in the wardrobe – it's gone everywhere with me for years now – but now I know I'll get back into it. I've lost 16 pounds [7 kilos] and I'm thrilled.'

Tania, thirty-five, has her own jewellery business in London

'I really am the last of the terrible eaters. I sit all day designing jewellery and have a coke and a bun on the go all the time. I get tired a lot and I work long hours, so I'm sometimes still picking after midnight.

'This diet made me want to go for it. I know it isn't the diet which does the work, it's you, but that has always been my downfall – lack of willpower. For the first time in my life I have stuck at something for six weeks and I feel it's part of my life now. I liked the way I could choose my own meals or follow the suggestions, and I did both. Being a picky eater and a lousy cook, I was glad to have lists of day-to-day meals I could choose, like beans on toast or omelettes, and not have to worry too much about mixing this with that. I just deducted carbograms which takes seconds.

'I also go home now and have a walk without fail. I take a lunch break and have a walk then too. I never eat absent-mindedly. I make a time to stop, and I stop, even if it's only for fifteen minutes. I never knew about sugar and the amounts in the food you buy, and I've become a bit of a Sherlock Holmes on the quiet now – checking labels and boring everyone with my knowledge! My tiredness has completely vanished and I'm working a lot more efficiently. This has been the big breakthrough.

'I lost 11 pounds [5 kilos], and the best part has been getting back into some particularly sexy black trousers which I love. It's really cheered me up.'

Lucy is nineteen and a hairdresser from Cheltenham

'I've lost over a stone [6 kilos] for my wedding. What I can't believe is that I've stopped thinking I need to weigh myself five times a day, which I never thought possible. I simply don't care about what I weigh any more, because I look slim and I feel slim, and that's all that matters. I have learned to understand carbograms and Monica is right – after a couple of weeks I didn't need to look anything up because I'd come to know the calories in what I myself ate. I'm not fixated, and I'll have a cake if I want one now. The only thing is that now, I *don't* want one!

'I was really keen to get back into my favourite jeans for my new life as a married woman. They're a really great fit and I couldn't believe it when the zip went up easily. It was all in my bottom, and I've lost it!'

FOOD FILE

All foods and meals have different carbohydrate (carbogram) values according to the size and manufacturer. For example, I have found five different values for a Bourbon biscuit! The menus in this book are averaged out, but here is a rough guide to standard foods and their carbohydrate ratings. Do not try to compare them with my diet menus. However, they are useful when you come across something you might never have eaten before, or are suddenly faced with an unfamiliar meal. It will become very useful to you to know carbograms off the top of your head!

BREADS AND CRACKERS

Ryvita Multigrain (slice)	6.0cg
1 slice white bread	17.0cg
1 slice wholemeal bread	17.0cg
Submarine roll	52.0cg
1 slice super-toasty bread (extra-thick)	25.0cg
1 slice thick bread	20.0cg
1 slice medium bread	17.0cg
1 wholemeal bap	28.0cg
1 bran biscuit	8.0cg
1 medium slice wholemeal	12.0cg
1 small thin slice wholemeal	9.0cg
1 slice gluten-free	9.0cg
1 slice malt wheatbread	16.0cg
1 baguette	35.0cg
1 bagel	43.0cg
1 pitta bread	43.0cg
1 naan	80.0cg
1 oatcake	8.0cg
1 piece French bread	22.0cg
1 English muffin	33.0cg

1 croissant	23.0cg
1 crumpet	17.0cg
1 crispbread	7.0cg
1 soft white roll	23.0cg
1 cream cracker	6.0cg
25g flour	18.0cg

BREAKFAST CEREALS

All these cereals have approx. 20cg per 30g serving.

All Bran
Shredded Wheat
Special K
Weetabix
Porridge oats
Sugar-free muesli
Grape Nuts

CHEESE

Cheese has no carbohydrates with the exception of
100g cottage cheese 3cg

EGGS

Eggs have almost no carbohydrate or sugar.

FATS

Fats have little carbohydrate or sugar with these exceptions:

Garlic butter	2.0cg
Healthy-eating lowest ever	6.0cg
Olive oil spread	1.0cg

FISH

Fish has no carbohydrate or sugar unless coated in breadcrumbs.

TINNED FRUIT IN JUICE (per 100g)

Apricot halves	10.0cg
Fruit cocktail	11.0cg
Grapefruit segments	10.0cg
Prunes	22.0cg
Mandarin oranges	8.0cg
Mixed fruit	14.0cg
Orange segments	11.0cg
Peach halves and slices	10.0cg
Pear halves and quarters	11.0cg
Pineapple cubes and rings	12.0cg
Raspberries	7.0cg
Strawberries	9.0cg

DRIED FRUIT

(Not recommended on this diet, but useful for essential high energy.)

1 apricot	3.0cg
1 tbsp raisins	18.0cg
1 fig	5.2cg
1 tbsp mixed dried fruit	21.0cg
6 prunes, stewed	6.0cg
1 tbsp sultanas	21.0cg

FRESH FRUIT

You must have the equivalent of FOUR pieces of fresh fruit every day. Fruit is important in every person's diet because it supplies fibre, water and micronutrients which are some of the most valuable cancer-fighting, immunity-boosting nutrients you can eat. Never get your immunity, vitamins or minerals from a bottle of pills. Your four choices can be a two-fruit salad, a glass of fresh fruit juice, a banana, a portion of berries like strawberries, raspberries, etc., or just four single items of fresh fruit – it doesn't matter, but it is vital that these are included every day. I have given you some idea of choices in the foods listed in The Diet section starting on page 71.

1 apple	11.0cg
banana	23.0cg
100g blackcurrants	21.0cg
50g black grapes	13.0cg
50g white grapes	15.0cg
1 lemon	0.6cg
2 slices mango	6.0cg
1 plum	5.0cg
1 orange	14.0cg
1 large slice pineapple	8.0cg
20g raspberries	3.0cg
20g strawberries	6.0cg

FRESH MEAT
Chicken, Turkey, Goose and Duck contain no carbohydrates or sugars.

MILK

Small can evaporated milk	14.0cg
¼ litre full-cream whole milk	14.0cg
¼ litre healthy-eating half-fat milk	14.0cg
¼ litre virtually fat-free skimmed milk	15.0cg
¼ litre soya milk, unsweetened	2.3cg

NUTS
Most nuts have about 1g of carbohydrate per handful.

OFFAL
Contains no carbohydrates or sugars.

OILS
Contain no carbohydrates or sugars.

PASTA (per 100g)
Only eat wholewheat pasta. When you eat pasta, you will need to calculate 60cg per 100g portion (this is about 4 tbsp).

RICE
Allow 60cg for every average serving of 4–5 tbsp rice.

SOUPS
These vary according to the make, but these are average carbogram values for 200ml:

Spinach soup	9cg
Chicken soup	15cg
Tomato soup	15cg
Carrot and coriander soup	8cg
Leek and potato soup	17cg

VEGETABLES
Vegetables are low in carbograms, so you can eat quite large portions of standard greens, salad vegetable and carrots without ruining your carbogram budget. Peas, beans and lentils are slightly higher in carbograms, but do not let this put you off eating them as they are essential in any diet.

3 tbsp most tinned baked beans	15.0cg
3 tbsp broad beans	14.0cg
3 tbsp Brussels sprouts, boiled	3.0cg
1 corn on the cob	14.0cg
⅙ white cabbage	4.0cg
1 carrot, raw	5.0cg
1 carrot, boiled	3.0cg

2 tbsp carrots	5.0cg
1 portion cauliflower, boiled	2.0cg
1 portion chips (chip shop)	64.0cg
1 courgette	2.0cg
2 tbsp of most green vegetables	2.0cg
2 tbsp leeks, boiled	2.0cg
60g mushrooms	less than 1cg
2 tbsp parsnips, boiled	5.0cg
½ green pepper	2.0cg
½ red pepper	5.0cg
1 medium potato, baked, plain	57.0cg
2 small potatoes, roast	52.0cg
1 portion ratatouille	7.0cg
Salad greens with cucumber	2.0cg
Full mixed salad, with tomato, no dressing	8.0cg
Spinach, boiled	0.7cg
2 tbsp swede, boiled	2.0cg
1 tbsp sweetcorn, tinned	0.6cg
1 tomato, fresh	2.0cg
Large tin tomatoes	6.0cg
1 bunch watercress	0.1cg
1 medium-sized yam	43.0cg

SAUCES AND DRESSINGS

1 tbsp bread sauce	6cg
1 tbsp brown sauce	3cg
2 tbsp cheese sauce	6cg
1 small can chicken soup	14cg
1 tsp chutney	4cg
1 tbsp cranberry sauce	12cg
2 tbsp tinned curry sauce	10cg
1 tbsp French dressing	0.7cg
1 tbsp Thousand Island dressing	4cg

1 portion hummus	7cg
1 tsp sweet chutney	5cg
1 tsp jam or marmalade	5cg
1 Oxo cube	0.8cg
Average amount peanut butter spread on bread	3cg
Small pub portion sweet pickle	7cg
1 tbsp salad cream	5cg
1 dsp relish in a burger	4cg
1 portion sweet and sour sauce	16cg
Small sachet tartare sauce	2cg
Sachet tomato ketchup	4cg
Tin tomato soup	18cg
Tin vegetable soup	30cg

DRINKS

Pint bitter	13cg
Pint dry cider	15cg
Pint sweet cider	25cg
Pint vintage cider	42cg
Pint lager	14cg
Pint low-alcohol lager	9cg
1 measure cream liqueur	6cg
1 measure clear liqueur	8cg
Sweet sherry	3cg
1 measure spirits	Trace cg
1 glass champagne	2cg
1 glass rosé wine	3cg
1 glass red wine	0.3cg
1 glass sparkling white wine	6cg
1 glass dry white wine	0.8cg
1 glass medium white wine	4cg
1 glass sweet white wine	7cg
1 glass blackcurrant squash	21cg

200ml apple juice	16cg
Standard-sized Coca-Cola	35cg
Can carbonated fruit juice drink	34cg
1 can lemonade	19cg
1 can Lucozade	40cg
200ml tomato juice	5cg
200ml pure orange juice	18cg
200ml pure grapefruit juice	15cg
Cup of coffee with milk, no sugar	1.3cg
Cup of drinking chocolate made with milk, no sugar	27cg
Cup of Horlicks made with milk, no sugar	33cg
Milk shake made from powder	22cg
1 bottle flavoured milkshake	53cg
Cup of Ovaltine with milk, no sugar	33cg
Cup of tea with milk, no sugar	1cg

SNACKS

Snack foods are discouraged, but here are some values so you
know how many precious carbograms you are squandering!

Standard packet crisps	16cg
Standard packet crisps, low-fat	19cg
Standard bag Doritos	22cg
25g Twiglets	15cg

COMPOSITE MEALS OUT

Danish pastry	56cg
Full English cooked breakfast (with cornflakes, toast and marmalade)	128cg
McDonald's bacon and egg McMuffin	27cg
McDonald's Big Breakfast	41cg
McDonald's hotcakes, butter and syrup, and sausage	82cg
Cornish pasty	45cg

Hot Dog	31cg
Ploughman's with cheddar cheese	83cg
Pork pie	35cg
Jumbo sausage in French bread	75cg
Full Sunday lunch	135cg
Average Chinese (chicken with cashew nuts, boiled rice, peppers)	108cg
Cod and chips	84cg
Chicken korma, pilau rice, 2 poppadums	100cg
Burger King Double Whopper	51cg
Chicken, fries and coleslaw	50cg
Kentucky Dippers	15cg
Party food – sausage roll, French bread, crudités, sour cream dip, olives, crisps and nuts – 1,400 calories	73cg

Recipes for Success

Here are all the recipes for the menus I've suggested on pages 71–6. Combine them with your own favourite dishes – as long as you've made sure they are within your calorie limits – or follow whole plans through.

Recipes

The recipes planned in this chapter are organized alphabetically, as follows:

Baby Balti Vegetables

Serves 2

Carbograms per serving 48

Ingredients

8 small new potatoes

8 baby carrots

2 tbsp vegetable or corn oil

8 very small onions

1 tsp ginger paste

1 tsp garlic purée or 1 crushed
garlic clove

1 tsp chilli sauce

1 small tin (125g) chickpeas

8 small courgettes or 2 standard
courgettes, sliced

8 mangetouts

8 baby sweetcorn

8 cherry tomatoes

1 tsp dried and crushed chillies

2 tsp sesame seeds

Naan bread, to serve

Method

1 Bring a pan of water to the boil and add the potatoes and carrots. Boil for 5 minutes and drain.

2 Heat the oil in a large frying-pan or wok over a high heat. Add the onions and fry until golden brown.

3 Lower the heat and add the ginger paste, garlic purée or crushed garlic and chilli sauce.

4 Add the chickpeas and stir-fry for 2 minutes until all the moisture has been absorbed.

5 Next, add the cooked potatoes and carrots, plus the courgettes, mangetouts, baby sweetcorn and tomatoes. Stir constantly over the heat for a further 2 minutes.

6 Finally, add the crushed chillies, turn onto a serving plate and sprinkle with the sesame seeds. Serve with naan.

Baked Banana

Serves 2

Carbograms per serving 38

Ingredients

2 bananas, skinned

Juice from 2 oranges

1 measure Grand Marnier or
    Cointreau (optional)

2 tbsp half-fat fromage frais

Method

1 Preheat the oven to 200°C/400°F/Gas Mark 6.

2 Lay the bananas in a shallow, ovenproof dish. Pour over the orange juice and liqueur, if using.

3 Bake in the centre of the oven, uncovered, for 10–15 minutes.

4 Serve with fromage frais.

Baked Brie Ciabatta

Serves 4

Carbograms per serving 42

Use goat's cheese or a garlic and herb cream cheese as an alternative to the Brie.

Ingredients

3 large tomatoes, sliced

Seasoning, to taste

1 garlic clove, halved

2 ciabatta loaves, halved lengthways

175g young spinach leaves

½ tbsp olive oil

225g Brie, thinly sliced

Method

1 Preheat the grill to hot. Put the tomatoes onto a baking sheet and season with salt and freshly ground black pepper. Cook for 5 minutes until softened and hot.

2 Meanwhile, rub the cut edge of the garlic clove over the cut surface of the ciabatta, then cut each piece of the ciabatta into three portions.

3 Preheat the oven to 220°C/425°F/Gas 7. Toss the spinach leaves in the olive oil and use the mixture to cover eight of the ciabatta pieces.

4 Top with the Brie and tomatoes. Place the topped ciabatta in piles of two, then top with the remaining plain ciabatta to make four triple-deck sandwiches.

5 Place the sandwiches on a large baking sheet and bake for 6–8 minutes until the cheese has melted slightly. Serve immediately.

Beef Goulash

Serves 4

Carbograms per serving 8 (without rice)

Ingredients

1 tbsp oil	1 × 450g tin chopped tomatoes
450g best braising steak, cubed	225g mushrooms, sliced
1 onion, chopped	1 red pepper, sliced into rounds
1 clove garlic, crushed (optional)	1 tbsp paprika
1 tbsp cornflour	2 tbsp half-fat crème fraîche
300ml red wine	Seasoning, to taste
150ml plain water	Green vegetables and rice, to serve

Method

1 Preheat the oven to 170°C/325°F/Gas Mark 3.

2 Put the oil into a large frying-pan over a low heat and heat

until moderately hot, add the beef and turn quickly for about 2 minutes to 'seal' it, until brown on all sides.

3 Add the onion and garlic, and continue to fry gently until the onion is transparent.

4 Turn down the heat, add the cornflour and toss until the meat and onions are thoroughly coated.

5 Transfer to a large ovenproof casserole dish and add the red wine and water. Cover and place in the oven. Cook for 1 hour.

6 Remove from the oven and add the tinned tomatoes, mushrooms and red pepper. Cook for a further 1½ hours.

7 Test the meat by removing one cube and cutting into it. It should fall apart quite easily. If it is not ready, return to the oven for a further 30 minutes.

8 When ready, allow to cool slightly for 5 minutes, then add the paprika and stir in the crème fraîche. Season as necessary, and serve immediately with green vegetables and rice.

Bombay Potato Salad

Serves 2
Carbograms per serving 18

Ingredients

450g small new potatoes, scrubbed	Seasoning, to taste
½ tsp ground coriander	1 green chilli pepper, de-seeded and
½ tsp ground cumin	chopped (optional)
75ml Greek yoghurt	Sprigs of parsley, chopped, to garnish

Method

1 Cook the potatoes in boiling, salted water for 15–20 minutes until tender.

2 To make the dressing, whisk together the spices, yoghurt, salt and pepper.

3 Drain the potatoes, leave to cool very slightly and stir into the dressing. Leave to cool completely, then cover and refrigerate until 20 minutes before required.

4 Before serving, stir in the chilli. Garnish with parsley.

Bran Cake

Makes 10 slices Carbograms per slice 52

This cake is fat-free, sugar-free and egg-free. The sweetness comes from the heavy concentration of dried fruits and it has a wonderfully nutty flavour and texture from the walnuts, almonds and seeds

Ingredients

50g All Bran	100g walnuts
300ml skimmed milk	50g flaked almonds
200g sultanas	50g sesame seeds
Butter or margarine, for greasing	50g sunflower seeds
100g dried apricots, halved	100g white self-raising flour, sifted
2 tbsp sugar-free marmalade	

Method

1 Put the All Bran into a large mixing bowl and cover with the milk.

2 Add the sultanas and dried apricots and stir. Leave to soak for at least one hour.

3 Heat the oven to 180°C/350°F/Gas Mark 4 and grease and line a 450g loaf tin.

4 When the All Bran mixture has been thoroughly soaked and softened, add the marmalade and combine well. Add the nuts,

sesame seeds, sunflower seeds and flour. Stir well and turn into the loaf tin. Bake in the centre of the preheated oven for about 45 minutes or until a skewer inserted into the middle of the loaf comes out clean. If the loaf is not ready, return it to the oven for a further 15 minutes.

5 When cooked, allow to cool in the tin. Wrap in foil and store in a tin in a cool place. Keeps for about a week.

Cannelloni Stuffed with Spinach & Almonds

Serves 4

Carbograms per serving 70

Ingredients

Olive oil
12–16 sheets fresh cannelloni
900g frozen spinach, thawed
100g ground almonds
6 tbsp half-fat crème fraîche
Seasoning, to taste

55g Gruyère or Mozzarella cheese, grated
Butter, for greasing
55g Parmesan cheese, grated
Mixed green salad, to serve

Method

1 Preheat the oven to 150°C/300°F/Gas Mark 2.
2 In a large pan of boiling water with 2 tsp of the olive oil, cook the cannelloni following the instructions on the package. When cooked, drain and keep warm.
3 Squeeze out any excess water from the spinach and place it in a bowl. Add the almonds, 2 tbsp of the crème fraîche, seasoning and the Gruyère or Mozzarella cheese. Mix well to combine.
4 Take one sheet of the cannelloni and lay a portion of the

133

spinach mixture on top of it. Roll it up, tucking in the ends. Do the same for the remainder of the cannelloni and stuffing.

5 Butter an ovenproof dish. Place the cannelloni inside it, side by side, to fit snugly. Cover with the remaining 4 tbsp crème fraîche. Sprinkle with the Parmesan cheese and bake in the middle of the oven for about 20 minutes. Serve piping hot with a mixed green salad.

Caramelized Pear

Serves 2
Carbograms per serving 17

Ingredients

1 tsp butter
2 pears, peeled, cored and cut in half

2 tsp sugar
1 tsp five-spice powder
Low-fat fromage frais, to serve

Method

1 Melt the butter in a non-stick frying-pan. Add the pears, sugar and five-spice powder.

2 Heat through gently, stirring occasionally. When the fruit is tender and slightly caramelized, remove it with a slotted spoon and serve it on warmed serving plates with 1 tbsp of fromage frais per person.

Carrot and Orange Salad

Serves 2

Carbograms per serving 16

Ingredients

2 large oranges

2 medium carrots

Bunch watercress, washed

2 dsp standard French dressing

30g pine kernels or sunflower
    seeds, toasted

Method

1 Peel the oranges with a knife so that no pith is left. Slice horizontally into very thin slices.

2 Peel the carrots. Using a potato peeler, peel long thin 'ribbons' down the side of each carrot. It might take a few tries to perfect the procedure, alternatively you could use the slicing side of a standard grater.

3 Arrange bunches of watercress on plates, toss the combined orange slices and carrot ribbons in the French dressing and pile onto the watercress. Just before serving, sprinkle a small handful of toasted seeds on top of each salad.

This salad is delicious served with plain grilled chicken, poached white fish or plain crusty French bread.

Chilli Con Carne

Serves 4

Carbograms per serving 18

Ingredients

450g extra-lean mince

1½ tbsp vegetable oil

1 small onion, finely chopped

1 clove garlic, crushed

1 × 250g tin tomatoes, chopped
  with herbs

2 tbsp concentrated tomato paste

1 × 450g tin kidney beans

1 green chilli, de-seeded and cut into
  thin rounds

1 tsp hot or mild chilli powder, to taste

Seasoning, to taste

Plain boiled rice and green salad or
  vegetables, to serve

Method

1 In a large frying-pan, fry the mince without any added fat or
  oil until the fat runs clear. Drain and set the meat aside.

2 Heat the oil and gently sauté the onion until softened. Drain
  away any excess oil. Add the mince, garlic, tomatoes and
  tomato paste. Turn down the heat, cover the pan and simmer
  for 5 minutes.

3 Next, add the chilli, kidney beans and chilli powder, if liked,
  to the mince mixture. Stir and continue to simmer for a further
  10 minutes.

4 Check the seasoning and add salt and pepper, if necessary.
  Serve with a portion of plain boiled rice and a green salad or
  vegetables.

Courgette & Tomato Gratin

Serves 2

Carbograms per serving 23

Ingredients

28g butter

2 tbsp vegetable oil

675g courgettes, thinly sliced

1 medium onion, chopped

1 clove garlic, crushed (optional)

450g chopped, tinned tomatoes

Seasoning, to taste

50g soft fresh breadcrumbs, mixed with a handful of dried herbs

28g Cheddar cheese, grated

Jacket potatoes or grilled chicken, to serve

Method

1 Preheat the oven to 200°C/400°F/Gas Mark 6.

2 Melt half the butter with 1 tbsp of the oil in a large saucepan over medium heat, add the courgettes, cover and cook for 5 minutes.

3 Heat the remaining oil in another medium-sized pan, add the onion, cover and cook for 5 minutes, stirring occasionally. Add the garlic and cook for a further 2 minutes.

4 Reduce the heat under the pan containing the onions, add the tomatoes, cover and cook for 5 minutes. Season well with salt and pepper.

5 Stir the courgettes into the tomato mixture and pour into a shallow, well-greased ovenproof dish. Level the top, sprinkle with the breadcrumbs and cheese, and dot with the remaining butter.

6 Bake, uncovered, for about 25–30 minutes until the top is golden brown and crisp. Serve with jacket potatoes or grilled chicken.

Feta & Walnut Salad

Serves 4

Carbograms per serving 12

This simple hot salad makes a light supper.

Ingredients

350g baby new potatoes or cubed
   old potatoes
2 tbsp vegetable oil
115g baby corn, halved lengthways
100g tinned broad beans
Salad leaves

50g walnuts, chopped
Grated peel of one orange
350g feta cheese, cubed
3 tbsp parsley, roughly chopped
Warm walnut bread, to serve

Method

1 Boil the potatoes for about 10 minutes or until done. Drain and reserve. If using the whole new potatoes, slice into rounds.
2 In a large frying-pan, heat the oil. Add the baby corn, broad beans and potato slices or cubes. Stir-fry the vegetables and beans in the oil over a medium heat for 3 minutes, browning the potatoes.
3 Line a dinner plate with a bed of salad leaves.
4 Add the chopped walnuts to the mixture in the frying-pan and heat through. Then add the grated orange peel.
5 Remove the pan from the heat, quickly add the feta cheese cubes and combine. Turn onto the salad leaves, garnish with chopped parsley and serve immediately with warm walnut bread.

Fresh Fruit Salad

Serves 4

Carbograms per serving 34

Ingredients

2 bananas

2 apples, washed

Juice of one lemon

1 grapefruit

40 seedless grapes, washed

100g fresh pineapple segments

100g blueberries, washed

Other fresh fruit in season, eg
    strawberries, raspberries

Juice of two oranges

Method

1 Peel and slice the bananas. Core and slice the apples, leaving the skins on. Place in a bowl with the lemon juice, and turn to coat well.

2 Halve the grapefruit and, using a grapefruit knife, remove the half-segments cleanly. Discard any pips, but take care to keep all the juice. Add to the bananas and apples.

3 Halve the grapes (leave the skins on) and add, along with the pineapple segments, blueberries and any other fruits.

4 Pour over the juice of the two oranges. Mix well and refrigerate before serving. Serve with 1 tbsp half-fat crème fraîche (optional).

Home-made Fresh Vegetable Soup

Serves 4

Carbograms per serving 26

Ingredients

225g ripe tomatoes
1 tbsp vegetable oil
1 medium onion, finely chopped
2 medium carrots, chopped
4–6 cauliflower florets
Handful French or runner beans,
 stringed

2 large potatoes, peeled and cut into
 small dice
1 bay leaf
½ tsp ground coriander
450ml vegetable stock
Salt and freshly ground black pepper
50ml low-fat crème fraîche

Method

1 Cut a cross in each tomato and immerse in boiling water for 30 seconds. Dip briefly into cold water, then remove and slip off the skins. Chop into quarters.

2 Heat the oil in a non-stick frying-pan and add the onion. Stir over a medium heat until soft. Transfer the onion to a saucepan and add the carrots, cauliflower, beans, potatoes and tomatoes. Add the bay leaf, coriander, stock, a little salt and plenty of black pepper. Cover and simmer for 20 minutes.

3 Allow the soup to cool a little, then remove the bay leaf and transfer the soup to a blender. If desired, reserve a few vegetables to serve as garnish in the soup. Adjust the seasoning and reheat, swirling the crème fraîche into the soup just before serving.

Hot Spiced Oranges

Serves 2

Carbograms per serving 14

Ingredients

2 large oranges, peeled and cut
into segments
1 tsp butter
1 measure Cointreau
Juice and zest of two more oranges

6 cloves
½ tsp cinnamon
2 tsp sugar
Fromage frais, to decorate

Method

1 Preheat the oven to 200°C/400°F/Gas Mark 6.
2 In a buttered, shallow ovenproof dish, place the orange segments and pour the Cointreau and orange juice over the top. Stir in half of the orange zest, and add the cloves and cinnamon. Sprinkle with sugar.
3 Cover the dish with foil and bake in the oven for 15–20 minutes.
4 Remove the dish from the oven, serve in individual bowls and decorate with a sprinkling of orange zest and fromage frais.

Kedgeree

Serves 2

Carbograms per serving 37

Ingredients

450g smoked haddock fillets
150ml skimmed milk, for poaching
100g Basmati rice
8g butter
½ onion, finely chopped
1–2 tsp curry powder
1 tsp ground turmeric

2 hard-boiled eggs, chopped
Seasoning, to taste
A handful of fresh parsley,
 chopped, to garnish
Crusty French bread or watercress
 salad, to serve

Method

1 Place the haddock in a large frying-pan and cover with milk. Poach gently for 10 minutes until cooked through. Remove the fish and set aside. Reserve the milk in the pan.

2 Meanwhile, set the rice to boil according to the instructions on the packet. When ready, drain and reserve.

3 In another frying-pan, gently sauté the onion in the butter. Add the cooked rice, curry powder and turmeric, and stir well until incorporated. Pour the reserved milk into the mixture and heat gently.

4 Flake the cooked haddock into large pieces and add to the rice mixture. Add the hard-boiled eggs and turn onto a warm serving dish.

5 Garnish with parsley, adjust the seasoning and serve hot, with crusty French bread or a watercress salad.

Lasagne Verde

Serves 4

Carbograms per serving 68

Ingredients

1 tbsp oil
10–12 sheets lasagne
680g leaf spinach
28g butter
Seasoning, to taste
Butter, for greasing
1 carton half-fat crème fraîche

225g Sage Derby cheese, grated
30g fresh white breadcrumbs
115g fresh Parmesan cheese, grated
30g parsley, chopped
Green salad, to serve

Method

1 Fill a saucepan half full of boiling water and 1 tbsp of oil, and cook the lasagne until soft. Drain.

2 Remove the stalks from the spinach and cook in the butter for about 5 minutes until soft. Remove from the heat and season with salt and pepper.

3 Pre-heat the oven to 190°C/375°F/Gas Mark 5.

4 Butter a large ovenproof dish and line the bottom and sides with half the lasagne. Cover with half the spinach mixture, half the crème fraîche and a final layer of lasagne.

5 Next, cover the final layer of lasagne with the remaining crème fraîche, Sage Derby cheese, breadcrumbs and Parmesan cheese.

6 Bake in the oven for 40 minutes. Garnish with parsley and serve immediately with a green salad.

Lentil Roast

Serves 2

Carbograms per serving 66

Ingredients

225g red or brown lentils, washed (soak brown lentils overnight)
60g butter
1 large onion, chopped
3 tomatoes, chopped
60g cornflakes, crushed
115g Cheddar cheese, grated
Salt and pepper
Mixed herbs, parsley and celery salt, to taste

Method

1 Heat oven to 180°C/350°F/Gas Mark 4. Grease a 1½ pint loaf tin.
2 Drain the lentils. Put them in a saucepan with ½ pint/285 ml water and bring to the boil. Cover the pan and reduce heat. Simmer until the lentils are soft and the water is absorbed.
3 In a frying-pan, fry the onion in the butter until soft but not brown. Add the tomatoes and cook for 5 minutes. Mash the lentils, add the cornflakes, the onion mixture and the remaining ingredients. Adjust the seasoning.
4 Turn into the loaf tin and sprinkle with a little more grated cheese. Bake for 30 minutes. Serve with a mixed salad or fresh steamed vegetables.

Lentil & Tofu Stir-fry

Serves 2

Carbograms per serving 21 (without rice)

Ingredients

3 tbsp soy sauce

3 tbsp sherry

1 garlic clove, crushed

Small piece root ginger, grated

250g tofu, cubed

4 tsp sesame oil

2 courgettes, cut into matchsticks

100g mushrooms, sliced

1 × 400g tin green lentils, drained

Seasoning, to taste

Boiled rice, to serve

Method

1 Mix together the soy sauce, sherry, garlic and ginger in a bowl. Add the tofu and stir until coated. Leave to marinate for about 10 minutes.

2 Heat half the sesame oil in a large frying-pan. Drain the tofu, reserving the marinade, and fry for 5 minutes until golden. Remove and keep hot.

3 Heat the remaining oil, add the vegetables and stir-fry. Add the lentils, tofu and reserved marinade, and cook for a further 3 minutes. Season and serve with boiled rice.

Mango or Orange or Raspberry & Rhubarb Sorbet

Serves 4

Carbograms per serving 30

Ingredients

4 mangoes or 4 oranges or 225g
   raspberries and 225g rhubarb

4 egg whites

56g caster sugar

Method

1 For Mango Sorbet, peel the mangoes and slice the flesh away from the core. Mash in a bowl or liquidize for 30 seconds until pulped.

   If you are making Orange Sorbet, remove the zest from the oranges and extract the juice. Mix both together in a medium-sized bowl.

   For Raspberry & Rhubarb Sorbet, peel the rhubarb and remove the stalks from the raspberries. Chop the rhubarb and put it into a pan with the raspberries and 1 tbsp water to prevent burning. Simmer until the fruit is very soft, about 5 minutes. Leave to cool.

2 In a medium bowl, whisk the egg whites until stiff but not dry. Gradually add the sugar, 1 tbsp at a time, whisking between each spoonful. When all the sugar is added, continue whisking until the meringue forms stiff peaks.

3 Fold the meringue into your chosen fruit, being careful not to beat it. Slowly incorporate the two. Turn into a freezer container and freeze immediately.

4 Remove after 1 hour and stir the sorbet. Freeze for a further 2 hours and stir again. Remove from freezer 20 minutes before serving to soften slightly.

Pasta Twists with Pesto and Nut Dressing

Serves 4

Carbograms per serving 49

Ingredients

200g fresh pasta twists, ideally multicoloured (white, red and green) (you can buy multicoloured pasta twists in the dried pasta ranges)

500ml olive oil

100ml wine vinegar

1 tsp caster sugar

Salt and freshly ground black pepper

1 tsp Dijon mustard

2 tbsp green pesto sauce

100g pine-nut kernels, toasted

Large handful rocket leaves

Method

1 Cook the pasta according to the directions on the packet.

2 Meanwhile, prepare the dressing. In a bowl, combine the olive oil, vinegar, sugar, salt and pepper (to taste), mustard and pesto. Whisk together for a minute. Add the pine nuts and the rocket.

3 Turn the hot pasta into a very hot serving dish, add the sauce and combine quickly. Serve immediately on its own, or with plain chicken which has been cut into thin strips and stir-fried.

Alternatively, you can serve with toasted hazelnuts, walnuts or almond flakes.

Pear & Apple Charlotte

Serves 4

Carbograms per serving 65

Ingredients

1 tbsp water

350g baking apples, peeled and cut into chunks

350g pears, peeled and cut into chunks

30g soft brown sugar

2 tsp golden syrup

1 egg yolk, beaten

Butter, for greasing

Caster sugar, for dusting

1 small loaf sliced white bread, with the crusts cut off

28g butter, melted

Half-fat crème fraîche, to serve

Method

1 Put the water into a heavy-based pan, add the chunks of fruit and cook over a medium heat until soft.

2 Add the sugar and syrup. Remove from the heat and add the beaten egg.

3 Heat the oven to 220°C/425°F/Gas Mark 7. Lightly butter a Charlotte mould or 1.2 litre Pyrex dish and dust with a little caster sugar.

4 Cut the crustless bread into fingers and lightly dip them into the melted butter. Use the bread to line the sides of the mould or dish, making sure the bread overlaps slightly. Cut a circle the size of the bottom of the mould and line the base.

5 Fill the mould with the fruit and cover the top with another large circle of bread. Seal the joins with your fingers.

6 Cook the Charlotte for 10 minutes at the higher heat, then lower the temperature to 190°C/375°F/Gas Mark 5 for a further 40 minutes. Leave to cool first, then chill for about 4 hours. Serve with crème fraîche.

Poached Cod in Caper Sauce with Lime Rice

Serves 4

Carbograms per serving 24 (with rice 80)

Ingredients

4 skinless, boneless cod fillets
1 teacup skimmed milk, for warming, and about 2 tbsp for mixing with flour
Seasoning, to taste
1 tbsp plain flour
28g butter

1 tsp grated lemon zest
2 tbsp capers
2 tbsp chopped parsley
2 tbsp half-fat crème fraîche
100g long-grain rice
Grated zest of 2 limes
Broccoli and French beans, to serve

Method

1 Place the cod fillets in a large frying-pan, add the milk and season with salt and pepper. Cover and poach gently for about 10 minutes until the fish is cooked through. Remove the fish and set aside, reserving the milk.

2 Add the flour to the warm milk, mixing a little with cold milk first to form a smooth paste. Stir constantly and add the butter and lemon zest.

3 Stir in the capers, parsley and crème fraîche. Season to taste with salt and pepper.

4 Meanwhile, cook the rice according to the instructions on the packet. Drain, and stir the lime zest into the rice.

5 Spoon the rice onto a warm serving dish. Top with the cod and pour the sauce over the top. Serve with broccoli and French beans.

Quorn & Pepper Kebabs

Serves 2

Carbograms per serving 67

Ingredients

2 tbsp olive oil

Crushed sea salt

2 tsp dried chillies, crushed

450g Quorn, cubed

1 onion, cut into quarters

1 red, 1 green and 1 yellow pepper

900g broccoli, steamed and puréed

100g Basmati rice, steamed

Method

1 Heat a barbecue or grill until hot. In a bowl, combine the oil, sea salt and chillies. Add the Quorn and leave to marinate for 10 minutes.

2 Separate the layers of onion so that they form large pieces. Cut each pepper into 4 large pieces.

3 Start to load the ingredients onto skewers, alternating with Quorn, red pepper, onion, green pepper, Quorn, and so on, until all the ingredients are equally divided between the 4 skewers.

4 Spoon the remaining marinade over the kebabs, turning so that all the sides are coated. Make sure that the surfaces are covered with chillies.

5 Place on a rack over a grill pan and grill, turning frequently, until golden brown or chargrilled. Serve immediately on hot plates on a bed of hot broccoli purée with steamed rice.

Red Bean & Tomato Curry

Serves 4

Carbograms per serving 5

Ingredients

2 tbsp sunflower oil
1 large onion, sliced
5 garlic cloves, crushed
1–2 fresh green chillies, cored, seeded and sliced
2.5cm (1in) piece of fresh root ginger, peeled and chopped
1 tsp curry powder

A pinch of cayenne pepper
Salt
½ tsp ground coriander
1 tsp turmeric
1 × 400g can chopped tomatoes
600g canned kidney beans
1 tbsp lemon juice
Fresh coriander leaves, to garnish

Method

1 Heat the sunflower oil in a large frying-pan, add the onion and garlic, chillies and ginger, and cook, stirring occasionally, until the onion is softened but not coloured.

2 Add the curry powder, cayenne pepper, salt to taste, ground coriander and turmeric and cook, stirring, for 2 minutes.

3 Add the tomatoes and most of their juice, and cook for about 3 minutes. Add the beans and cook for a further 5 minutes.

4 Add the lemon juice and serve hot, garnished with coriander leaves.

Roast Pineapple

Serves 4

Carbograms per slice 10

Ingredients

1 whole pineapple

8 star anise

Half-fat crème fraîche or fromage frais, to serve

Method

1 Preheat the oven to 200°C/400°F/Gas Mark 6. Peel the pineapple and remove the central hard core. Alternatively, buy a whole fresh pineapple which is ready-prepared.

2 Stud the pineapple all over with the star anise. Cover tightly with foil and roast in the centre of the oven for 30 minutes.

3 Remove the pineapple from the oven and cut into large, 5-cm rings. Serve immediately with crème fraîche or fromage frais.

Salade Niçoise

Serves 2

Carbograms per serving 35

Ingredients

2 tbsp olive oil

1 tbsp wine vinegar

2 leaves fresh mint, roughly crushed

Salad greens

8 small, waxy new potatoes, scrubbed, boiled and cooled

1 small tin tuna fish in brine, drained

100g French beans, steamed for 5 minutes and cooled

Small handful of black olives

2 hard-boiled eggs, shelled

Ground black pepper, to taste

Method

1 In a small jug, combine the oil and vinegar and add the mint leaves.

2 Arrange the salad greens on a serving plate, top with the potatoes, tuna and beans, then scatter the olives over the top. Quarter each hard-boiled egg and add to the salad.

3 Remove the mint from the dressing and pour over the salad just before serving. Season with black pepper.

Salmon Mousseline with Fresh Tomato Sauce

Serves 4

Carbograms per serving 20

Ingredients

300g salmon fillet, skinned and cubed
1 clove garlic, chopped
1 egg
1 egg white
Seasoning, to taste
4 large tbsp half-fat crème fraîche
Butter, for greasing

Sauce
350g tomatoes, peeled and chopped
2 tbsp half-fat crème fraîche
2 tsp lemon juice
1 tbsp chopped dill
Sprig of dill, to garnish
French toast, to serve

Method

1 Preheat the oven to 180°C/350°F/Gas Mark 4. Place a roasting pan half full of very hot water into the oven.

2 Purée the salmon and garlic in a blender for 1 minute. Add the egg and egg white. Season, then mix again for a few seconds, then add the crème fraîche. Mix once again, but stop as soon as the mixture is thick and smooth. Leave to chill in the refrigerator.

3 Generously grease a 600-ml terrine or loaf tin. Spoon the mousseline inside and cover with a piece of greased foil. Place the terrine or tin inside the water bath and bake for 35 minutes or until the top is firm. Allow to cool.

4 Meanwhile, make the sauce by combining all the ingredients. Turn the mousseline out onto a serving dish and slice. Pour the sauce around each slice.

5 Serve garnished with a sprig of dill, accompanied by freshly made thin French toast.

Smoked Salmon & Avocado Salad

Serves 2

Carbograms per serving 3

Ingredients

Salad greens	1 avocado pear
Fresh vinaigrette dressing	Juice and zest of one lime
2 slices smoked salmon	

Method

1 Place the salad greens onto a serving plate. Drizzle vinaigrette over the top. Slice the smoked salmon into thin strips and pile on top of the greens.

2 Peel the avocado pear and halve, removing the stone. Place one half stone-side down on a plate and slice horizontally. Gently press the avocado to one side so that it fans out. Repeat with the other avocado half.

3 Balance the avocado slices on top of the salmon, pour over the lime juice and garnish with a sprinkling of lime zest.

Smoked Salmon on Potato Cakes

Serves 2

Carbograms per serving 30

Ingredients

225g old potatoes, peeled
1 egg, beaten
100ml skimmed milk
Seasoning, to taste
2 tbsp white flour
8g butter, melted, and butter for
  greasing

Squeeze of lemon juice
2 slices smoked salmon
2 tbsp half-fat crème fraîche
A handful of chopped, fresh
  parsley

Method

1 Preheat the oven to 200°C/400°F/Gas Mark 6.
2 Boil and simmer the potatoes for about 20 minutes until done and then drain.
3 Add the egg and milk and mash well. Season and add the flour and use your hands to shape the mixture into 4 large potato balls.
4 Grease a baking sheet, and place the potato balls on it, flattening them to make large cakes. Brush with melted butter and bake in the centre of the oven for 25 minutes.
5 Meanwhile, cut the smoked salmon pieces into thin strips and toss in the lemon juice.
6 When the potato cakes are ready, remove from the oven and allow to cool slightly for 5 minutes. Divide the smoked salmon pieces between the four cakes and pile on top. Spoon 2–3 teaspoonsful of crème fraîche over the smoked salmon in mounds and top with a sprinkling of fresh parsley.

Spaghetti with Smoked Salmon & Dill

Serves 2

Carbograms per serving 62

Ingredients

125g fresh spaghetti
2 tsp olive oil
1 clove garlic, crushed
50g smoked salmon, cut into strips
Seasoning, to taste

2 tbsp half-fat crème fraîche
1 fresh frond of dill, snipped, and
   one frond to garnish
Chopped fresh parsley, to garnish

Method

1 Cook the spaghetti in a pan of boiling water for 3 minutes or as directed on the package. Drain.

2 Heat the oil in a large frying-pan. Add the garlic and salmon, and cook for 30 seconds, stirring constantly.

3 Add the drained cooked spaghetti to the pan, heat through and season to taste.

4 Just before serving, add the crème fraîche and dill, and stir through quickly but do not apply heat. Turn straight onto hot plates, sprinkle with parsley and garnish with dill.

Note: This dish goes cold very quickly, so hot plates are essential.

Spiced Vegetable Risotto
with Green Lentils

Serves 4

Carbograms per serving 71

Ingredients

100g dried green lentils	340g rice
1 large aubergine	150ml white wine or vermouth
2 courgettes	900ml boiling water
4 tbsp olive oil	2 tbsp green peppercorns
1 tsp each: cumin, coriander seeds,	28g butter
paprika and garam masala	50g fresh Parmesan, grated from
2 onions, sliced	block
4 cloves garlic, crushed	

Method

1 Simmer the lentils for about 20 minutes until soft. Drain and reserve. Preheat oven to 190°C/375°F/Gas Mark 5.

2 Cut the aubergine and courgettes into cubes.

3 Heat the oil in a heavy ovenproof pan and sauté the spices. Add the lentils and fry over medium heat until slightly brown. Then add the aubergine, courgettes, onions and garlic, and cook gently for about 4 minutes or until soft.

4 Add the rice, wine or vermouth, boiling water and peppercorns. Place in the oven and bake until the rice is cooked through, about 45 minutes.

5 Before serving, gently stir in the butter and grated Parmesan.

Spicy Cajun Chicken

Serves 4

Carbograms per serving 2 (with rice 59)

Ingredients

4 tsp citrus pepper

4 tsp coriander seeds

4 tsp cayenne pepper

4 tsp dried garlic granules

4 tsp dried onion granules

4 tsp dried chillies

4 skinless, boneless chicken breasts, slightly flattened

3–4 tbsp olive oil

200g cooked rice or a selection of dressed salad leaves, to serve

Method

1 Combine all the spices and flavourings.

2 Lightly brush the chicken with oil. Press spice and flavourings mixture into the chicken breasts to cover all surfaces.

3 Heat the remaining oil in a large frying-pan. Add the chicken and sauté gently until cooked thoroughly, turning every few minutes. Turn up the heat and sear the chicken.

4 Serve immediately on hot rice, cutting the chicken breasts diagonally into thick slices. Alternatively, serve on a bed of dressed salad leaves.

Spicy Yoghurt-baked Chicken

Serves 2

Carbograms per serving 66

Ingredients

1 carton live, plain bio yoghurt
Juice of 1 fresh lime
A little fresh ginger root, grated
A few fennel seeds
1 tsp each: cumin, turmeric and
  cayenne pepper

1 clove garlic, crushed
2 skinless, boneless chicken
  breasts
125g Basmati rice
Green salad, to serve

Method

1 To prepare the marinade, combine the yoghurt, lime juice, ginger, fennel seeds, spices and garlic in a bowl and mix thoroughly.
2 Place the chicken in the marinade, coat completely, cover and set aside for 2–8 hours.
3 Preheat the oven to 180°C/350°F/Gas Mark 4. Remove the chicken from the marinade and place in an ovenproof dish, cover and bake in the oven for 25 minutes. Spread the marinade sauce over the chicken and return to the oven for a further 20 minutes.
4 Boil the rice as directed on the packet and drain. Serve the chicken on a bed of rice with a green salad.

Spinach & Avocado Salad

Serves 4

Carbograms per serving 5

Ingredients

450g young leaf spinach

2 ripe avocados

2 tbsp hazelnut oil

2 tsp wine vinegar

Seasoning, to taste

85g hazelnuts, coarsely chopped

Crusty French bread, to serve

Method

1 Remove the stalks from the spinach leaves, wash and pat dry.

2 Peel, stone and slice the avocados.

3 Mix the oil, vinegar and seasoning in a bowl. Add the avocados and spinach and sprinkle with hazelnuts.

4 Toss the salad lightly at the table, making sure that the avocado does not break up. Serve with crusty French bread.

Stir-fry Chicken with Carrot & Orange Salad

Serves 4

Carbograms per serving 7

Ingredients

2 skinless, boneless chicken breasts

2 tsp dried chillies

2 tbsp vegetable oil

Fresh watercress

2 oranges

2 carrots

Soy sauce, to taste

Method

1 Cut the chicken breasts into thin strips. Sprinkle the dried chillies onto a small plate and roll the chicken in them until lightly coated. Press the chicken into the chillies, if necessary, to make them stick.

2 Heat the oil in a large frying-pan and gently fry the chicken, turning quickly at first to seal. Cover the pan and lower the heat to cook the chicken.

3 Sprinkle watercress over a serving dish to cover the surface. Remove the zest from the oranges and reserve. Peel the oranges and cut into segments.

4 With a potato peeler, peel the carrots lengthwise to form long strips. (These should curl slightly to form 'ribbons'.) Combine with the orange segments and pile onto the watercress bed.

5 Check that the chicken is cooked by cutting into a strip of meat. The flesh should be white throughout without a hint of pink. Turn up the heat to brown.

6 Add the grated orange zest and a good dash of soy sauce. Combine well, then turn straight onto the top of the salad and serve immediately.

Strawberry & Cucumber Salad

Serves 4

Carbograms per serving 10

Ingredients

Lamb's lettuce or watercress
450g strawberries, hulled
1 whole cucumber, peeled
2 tbsp hazelnut oil

1 tbsp raspberry vinegar
A few mint leaves, crushed
Cold chicken or ham, to serve

Method

1 Line a decorative serving dish with lamb's lettuce or watercress.

2 Slice the strawberries very thinly and place them in a bowl.

3 Using the long-slice part of a grater, hold the cucumber so that it is facing downwards and grate long strips down its length to form 'ribbons'. Avoid the seeds in the middle of the cucumber and work round until only the seeds are left. Discard.

4 Combine the cucumber 'ribbons' with the strawberries and pile onto the watercress or lamb's lettuce.

5 Mix all the dressing ingredients together separately, including the mint leaves, shake well and leave to stand until just before serving. Discard the mint before pouring. Do not toss the salad. Serve with cold chicken or ham.

Sweet & Sour Vegetables with Rice

Serves 4

Carbograms per serving 67 (without rice 10)

Ingredients

4 tbsp vegetable oil	1 tbsp malt vinegar
1 onion, chopped finely	1 tbsp soy sauce
4 courgettes, sliced	1 tbsp each sultanas and almonds
100g French beans	1 tsp crushed cloves
8 baby sweetcorn	2 tbsp honey
200g mushrooms, sliced	Seasoning, to taste
2 carrots, chopped into batons	Boiled rice, to serve

Method

1 Heat the oil in a large frying-pan and cook the onion until soft. Add the rest of the vegetables and stir well. Cook for 5 minutes.

2 Add all the other ingredients, stir well and cook through for a further 3 minutes. Serve with boiled rice.

Szechuan Pepper & Tofu Stir-fry

Serves 4
Carbograms per serving 66

Ingredients

3 tbsp vegetable oil
1 × 285g pack tofu, drained and cut into cubes
1 tsp Chinese 5-spice powder
¼ tsp chilli powder
1 red pepper, de-seeded and cut into strips
1 bunch salad onions, trimmed and sliced diagonally

2 tsp cornflour
1 tbsp dark soy sauce
1 tbsp dry sherry
2 tbsp dark brown sugar
4 tbsp water
1 tsp sesame seeds, toasted
2 sheets egg noodles

Method

1 Heat 1 tbsp of the oil in a large frying-pan, add the tofu and fry for 1–2 minutes, until brown. Remove and drain.
2 In a bowl, mix the spices with the tofu. Heat the remaining oil, add the pepper and spring onions, and stir-fry.
3 Combine the cornflour, soy sauce, sherry, sugar and water, and add to the vegetables. Cook for a further 2 minutes, stirring until thickened.
4 Add the sesame seeds and the tofu to the vegetable mixture and heat gently for a further 1–2 minutes.
5 Cook the noodles according to the instructions on the package, drain and combine with the tofu mixture. Serve immediately on hot plates.

Tofu Sticks with Spicy Spinach

Serves 2

Carbograms per serving 15

Ingredients

1 tbsp vegetable oil

200g packet frozen spinach, thawed

1 green chilli, finely chopped

1 tsp chilli powder, plus a little for dusting

200g tofu, rinsed and cut into cubes

1 red and 1 green pepper, cut into quarters

8 slices onion, cut suitably for threading onto skewers

2 tsp sesame seeds, toasted

Salt and coarsely-ground black pepper

Method

1 Preheat grill or barbecue to hot.

2 Put 1 tbsp oil into a large frying-pan over a gentle heat and fry the spinach with the chopped chillies and the chilli powder for 1–2 minutes. Remove, drain and keep warm in an oven-proof dish.

3 Thread the tofu cubes, the pepper quarters and the onion onto two skewers, alternating them. Brush or drizzle over the other tbsp of oil, making sure all sides are coated.

4 Grill for 5 minutes, turning frequently and making sure the kebabs do not burn. Brush with any remaining or a little extra oil to prevent them drying out. Finally, dust with a little chilli powder before continuing to grill for a further minute.

5 Turn the kebabs onto the hot spinach mixture and sprinkle with the toasted sesame seeds to serve.

Two-Pear Salad

Serves 4

Carbograms per serving 4

This dish works best with chargrilled salmon or white fish, or large chargrilled prawns.

Ingredients

1 large, ripe dessert pear

1 large, ripe avocado pear

Juice of 1 lemon

2 tbsp olive oil

1 tbsp raspberry vinegar

1 tsp sugar

Coarsely ground black pepper

Method

1 Peel the pear, slice into quarters and remove the core. Slice carefully into thin slices.

2 Cut the avocado pear in two, remove the stone and peel each half. Cut into thin slices.

3 Interleave the slices on a round serving dish, alternating pear with avocado to form a wheel. Squeeze lemon juice over the top to prevent browning.

4 Mix the dressing ingredients together and, just before serving, drizzle over the top.

Waldorf Salad

Serves 2

Carbograms per serving 23

Ingredients

1 red apple, sliced

2 celery sticks, cut into 2-cm strips

20 grapes, halved

12 walnuts, crushed into pieces

1 tbsp good mayonnaise

Lettuce leaves

Method

1 Place the apple and celery in a bowl.

2 Add the grapes and walnuts. Bind with the mayonnaise and mix well.

3 Turn out onto the bed of lettuce on a serving plate and serve.

Warm Chicken Salad

Serves 2

Carbograms per serving 14

This is an incredibly quick and easy dish to make. It is low-calorie and full of goodness for any dieter. Have different spices at the ready to vary the taste.

Ingredients

Selection of dried spices or herbs, to taste

1 skinless, boneless chicken breast, cut into thin strips *or*

200g bought chicken strips, cut for stir-frying

Packet of bought Bistro-style or Nantaise salad (lamb's lettuce and grated beetroot)

½ carrot, grated

½ courgette, grated

1 tbsp sweetcorn

1 tbsp pine kernels (optional)

1 tbsp soy sauce (optional)

1 tbsp good-quality French dressing (not low-fat)

Method

1 Place 2 teaspoons of your chosen spice or herb mixture on a small plate. Roll the chicken pieces in them until they are coated evenly.

2 Arrange the salad on a serving plate. Make a bed of Salade Nantaise leaves and top with the carrot, courgette and sweetcorn.

3 Toast the pine kernels by placing them in a frying-pan with 1 teaspoon of oil and cook over a medium heat for several minutes. Cover the pan and keep shaking. Check when the pine kernels have turned brown and toasted, remove from the heat and turn out onto a kitchen towel. Reserve.

4 Heat the rest of the oil in a frying-pan and add the chicken pieces. Keep the heat low and turn several times until the chicken has turned white on the outside. Cover the pan and leave to cook for a further 5 minutes.

5 Turn up the heat to brown the chicken, add the soy sauce, if using, and flash fry for a further 1–2 minutes. Turn immediately onto the salad, dress with vinaigrette and toss the toasted pine kernels over the top to serve.

Winter Salad

Serves 4

Carbograms per serving 35

Ingredients

2 red apples, grated including skin
1 courgette, grated including peel
Juice of one lemon
Quarter of a white cabbage, finely chopped or grated
2 large carrots, peeled and grated

Quarter of a red cabbage, finely chopped or grated
50g dried sultanas
50g walnut pieces (optional)
4 tbsp vinaigrette
Jacket potatoes and cheese, to serve

Method

1 Put the apples and courgette into a bowl and squeeze lemon juice over them to prevent browning.

2 Add all the other vegetables, dried sultanas and walnuts, and mix well. Just before serving, add the vinaigrette and toss. Transfer to a salad bowl. Serve with jacket potatoes and cheese.